WEIGHT FREESTYLE COOKBOOK

2018 WEIGHT WATCHERS FREESTYLE RECIPES AND THE GUIDE TO LIVE HEALTHIER INCLUDE A 30 DAY MEAL PLAN FOR ULTIMATE WEIGHT LOSS

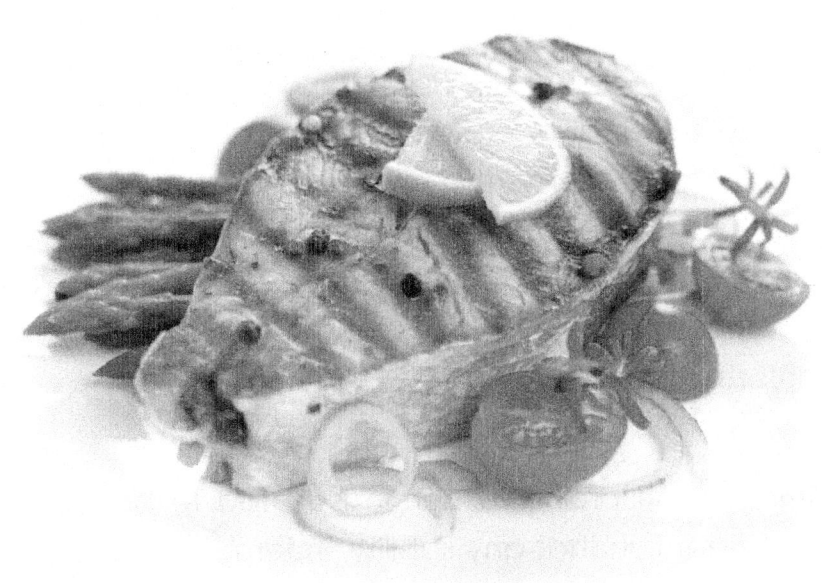

Anna Kaiser

@ Copyright 2017 by Anna Kaiser All rights reserved.

This document is geared towards providing exact and reliable information in regards to the topic and issue covered. The publication is sold with the idea that the publisher is not required to render accounting, officially permitted, or otherwise, qualified services. If advice is necessary, legal or professional, a practiced individual in the profession should be ordered.

- From a Declaration of Principles which was accepted and approved equally by a Committee of the American Bar Association and a Committee of Publishers and Associations.

In no way is it legal to reproduce, duplicate, or transmit any part of this document in either electronic means or in printed format. Recording of this publication is strictly prohibited and any storage of this document is not allowed unless with written permission from the publisher. All rights reserved.

The information provided herein is stated to be truthful and consistent, in that any liability, in terms of inattention or otherwise, by any usage or abuse of any policies, processes, or directions contained within is the solitary and utter responsibility of the recipient reader. Under no circumstances will any legal responsibility or blame be held against the publisher for any reparation, damages, or monetary loss due to the information herein, either directly or indirectly.

Respective authors own all copyrights not held by the publisher.

The information herein is offered for informational purposes solely, and is universal as so. The presentation of the information is without contract or any type of guarantee assurance.

The trademarks that are used are without any consent, and the publication of the trademark is without permission or backing by the trademark owner. All trademarks and brands within this book are for clarifying purposes only and are the owned by the owners themselves, not affiliated with this document.

TABLE OF CONTENTS

Introduction 9
    What is the Weight Watchers Diet? 10
    Basics of the Weight Watchers Plan 12
    Why Choose Weight Watchers? 16
    What Foods Can I Eat? 19
    Started with Weight Watchers 20
    What are the SmartPoints® 22

The Smart Points History 24
The benefits of the Smart Points 25
The negatives of Smart Points 26
Weight Watchers FreeStyle 2018 28
What's New Adding To The Program 28
What's Still Stay...30
Freestyle SmartPoints Recipes 34
Freestyle Butter Chicken Pot Pasta 35
Freestyle One Pot Garlicky Cuban Pork 37
Freestyle Pimento Chile Chicken..................................39
Freestyle White Chicken Chili..40
Freestyle Buffalo Wing Hummus...................................42
Freestyle Ham and Cheese Egg Cups 43
Freestyle Corn and Zucchini Summer Frittata 45
Turkey Meatball & Veggie Soup....................................47
Freestyle Shredded Mexican Chicken 49
Freestyle Baked Chicken Tenders 51
Freestyle The Best Turkey Chili 53
Freestyle Mexican Chicken Cauliflower.....................55
A 30 Day Meal Plan to Get You Started 57
Weight Watchers Breakfasts 63
Pancakes 64
Healthy Morning Cookies 65
Cinnamon Rolls 66
Mushroom and Spinach Quiche 67
Apple Muffin 68
Potato and Cheese Casserole 69

- Crispy Apple Surprise 70
- Breakfast Jelly Pudding – 71
- Pumpkin Muffins –.. 72
- Blackberry and Peach Smoothie 73
- Morning Burritos 74
- Breakfast Souffle 75
- Breakfast Bars –... 76
- French Toast –.. 77
- Cheese and Ham Omelet – 78
- Spiced Honey Cake 79
- Blueberry Muffins 80
- Yogurt Fluff – 81

Weight Watchers Lunches 82
- Creamy Pesto Pasta – 83
- BBQ Pork Sandwich 84
- Italian Chicken 85
- Baked Tortellini.. 86
- Cheesy Mushrooms 87
- Baked Burrito... 88
- Italian Bread with some Tuna Salad.............................. 89
- Turkey and Cheese Sandwich 90
- Veggie Soup 91
- Cheeseburger Soup 92
- Pasta Veggies... 93
- Bacon Wrap.. 94
- Baked Fish 95
- Beef Ziti Bake.. 96

- Chicken Salad 97
- Egg Salad 98
- Beef Burgers 99

Weight Watchers Dinners recipes 100
- Cheesy Chicken Chops 101
- Jalapeno Chicken 102
- Cilantro Lime Shrimp 103
- Spinach and Chicken Crescents 104
- Steak and Mashed Potatoes 105
- Honey Salmon 106
- Veggie Pork Chops 107
- Mexican Casserole 108
- Chicken Thai Wrap 109
- Pita Bread Pizza 110
- Potato Soup 111
- Roast Beef with Veggies 112
- Mushroom Steak 113
- Cheese and Tuna Sandwich – 114
- Cola Chicken 115
- Beef Chili 116
- Vegetable Quesadilla 117
- Baked Chicken – 118
- Chicken and Dumplings 119

Smart Points Slow Cooker Recipes 120
- Slow Cooked Beef and Barbeque 121
- Tasty Chicken Teriyaki 123
- Coconut Chicken Curry 124

Great Chicken Italiano 125
Smart Points Slow Cooker Tacos 126
One-Pot Chicken with Potatoes 128
Rosemary chicken with lemon 129
Chicken and Dumplings 130
Tortilla Soup with Chicken 132
Spicy Slow Cooker Chicken 133
Chicken Noodle Soup 134
Slow Cooked Pork Chili 135
Black Bean Enchiladas & Spinach 136
Pulled Pork and Cheese Sandwich 138
Zuppa Toscana Soup 139
Spicy Pulled Pork 140
Tender Beef Stroganoff 142
Tasty Beef Burgundy 143
Bean Soup with Pork Sausage 145
Slow Cooker Pork Pot Roast 146
Conclusion 147

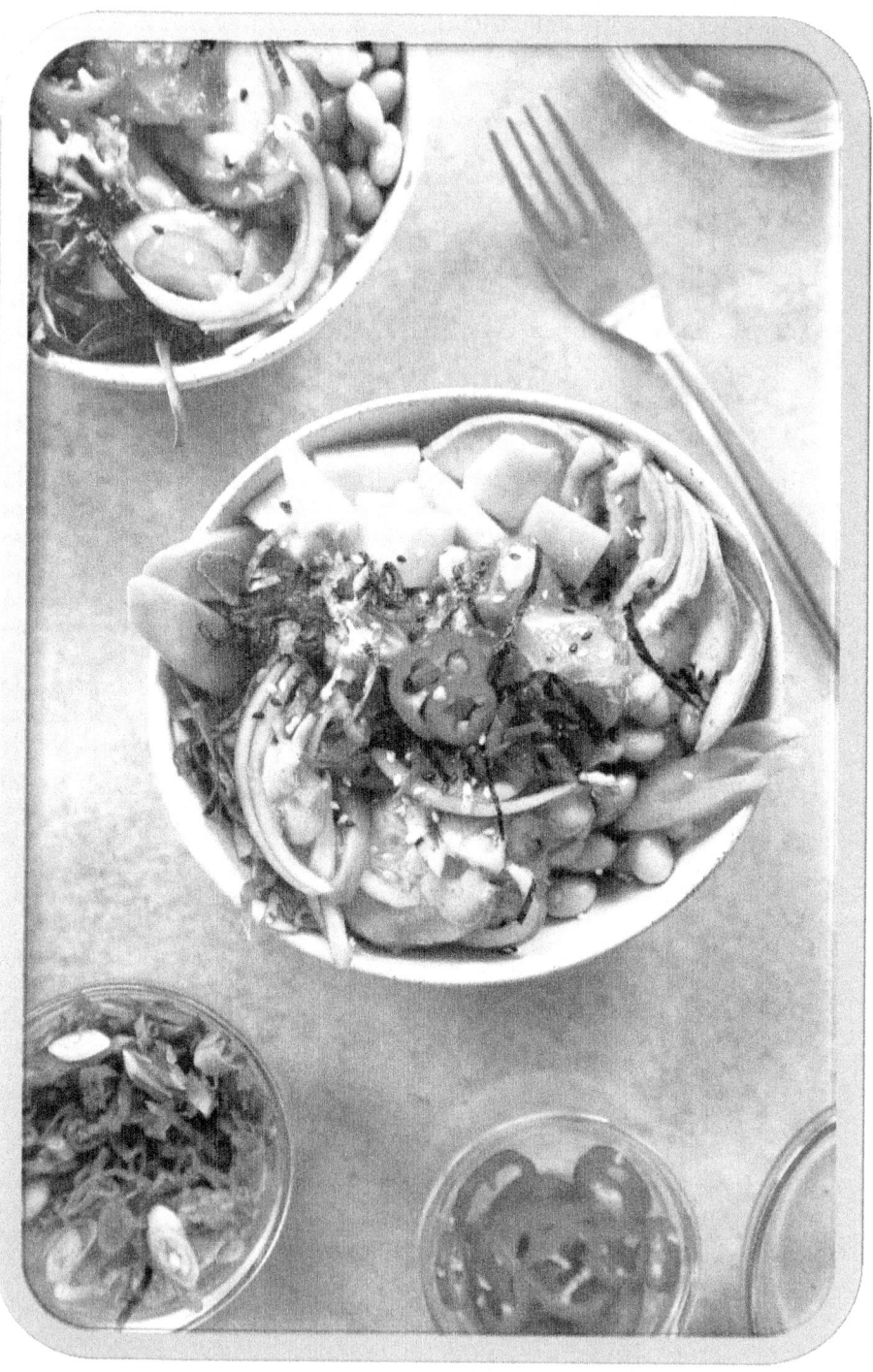

INTRODUCTION

When it comes to picking out the right diet plan that you are going to use, there are a lot of options that you can choose from. All of them are going to offer advice and suggestions on what you are able to do to lose weight, but many of them are unsafe, offer bad advice, and are just too hard to follow for the long term.

This guidebook is going to spend some time talking about the Weight Watchers plan, a plan that is going to help you to lose weight and get in better health for your whole life and not just for a few weeks. We are going to explore how to make this diet plan work the best for your needs.
We also include the latest update version of the latest Weight Watchers FreeStyle information and recipes to go with.
As more information and recipes updated I will be Able to write more on the complete all new freestyle cookbook in the near future.

When you are first looking to lose weight or get in better health than you were before, you will find that there are a lot of different weight loss plans that you are able to follow. Some are going to ask you to limit the types of certain foods that you are allowed to eat, some will limit the times that you are allowed to eat during the day, and some can be really unhealthy and unsafe (even if they do drop some of the pounds in the beginning). All of this information can be hard to sift through and you may feel worried that you are not able to find the right diet plan with the right rules that will work for you.

Most Americans are living an unhealthy lifestyle and because of this, there are a ton of weight loss and diet programs out there. Americans are eating more calories than ever, most of which are going to be full of saturated fats, sugars, and other things that are bad on the body. Add to this that most of these same people are going to live a sedentary lifestyle that includes sitting in front of the desk all of the time and then going home and just watching television all of the time. All of this is going to add together in order to make you feel unhealthy and gain a lot of weight in the process.

What is the Weight Watchers Diet?

Weight Watchers is one of the best diet plans that you can choose. It is not going to be as restrictive as some of the other diet plans that are out there. You are not going to have to pick whether you are allowed to eat grains or eating some fats in your diet. You will get to pick out the foods that you would like to eat, but you will be limited rather on the amount of points, known as SmartPoints® in this program, that you are allowed to eat each day. This makes it a little bit healthier to follow because you will be able to choose a lot of healthy and tasty foods, you won't be stuck eating foods that are unhealthy and bad for the body or having to feel like you are deprived all the time.

Let's take a look at this program a bit more. The idea behind Weight Watchers is to make you more conscious about the food choices that you are making. Many diet plans tell you to avoid this or that and then concentrate too much on the amount of calories that you are consuming. As long as you are staying in this calorie count, they promise that you are going to lose weight. The issue with this is that it isn't always about the amount of calories that you are eating as it is about the type of calories that you eat. 100 calories of fruit are much different than a 100 calories of a cookie and this is kind of how the Weight Watchers diet is going to focus on.

With the diet, you are going to be given a set amount of SmartPoints® that you are allowed to have each day and then you are able to have a few more during the week for when you want a cheat day or to eat out every once in a while. The amount of points that you are allowed will be based on your own personal profile. Depending on your height, current weight, and how much you would like to lose, you will be given an amount of SmartPoints® that you are able to use up each week.

Note: The SmartPoints® have been changed a bit in the last few years. In the past, participants were able to workout each day and then add in some more of the points each day. This started to develop an unhealthy relationship between working out and the foods that the participants were eating. While exercise is an important part of this whole process and can help you to keep healthy, it is not a good idea to think about food being the reward for the exercise that you do each day.

The foods that are healthier for you, such as healthy carbs, protein, and fruits and vegetables are going to be given fewer points, meaning that you are able to eat more of them. On the other hand, the foods that are considered bad, the ones that are full of sugars, saturated fats, and other bad things are going to have a higher point value for each serving. You are not forbidden from eating certain foods during this diet plan, but when you are faced on the choice of eating all your calories for the day in two pieces of cake or getting a few balanced meals, you are more likely to choose the latter.

One of the reasons that Weight Watchers is so much more effective than you will find with some of the other diet plans is because of the meetings. Not only are you going to concentrate on eating the right foods and trying to get in a bit more exercise and activity to your daily routine, you will also need to attend meetings. These meetings are where you will be held accountable for your weight loss and the choices that you make. You will have a private weigh-in each time that you go, feel encouraged to keep meeting your goals, and even hear stories and get advice on how to keep going.

Most people find that while these meetings are a bit intimidating in the beginning, they are going to make a big difference in the amount of weight that you will lose overall. You will be able to ask your questions, get advice, and find out whether you are staying on track of the diet plan or not.

In addition to eating the right kinds of foods, you will need to pay attention to the amount of exercise that you are getting each day. While you will not be able to get more points for food any longer when your workout, you will still need to add in some more exercise in order to work out the heart, lose more weight, and feel even better. Make sure to add in at least 30 minutes of moderate exercise most days of the week and you are going to feel so much better than you did in the past.

Basics of the Weight Watchers Plan

Weight Watchers is one of the best weight loss programs you can get on. It allows you to lose a lot of weight in a safe and effective way. While some of the other diet plans make a lot of promises along the way, most of them are hard to keep up or leave you feeling deprived for the long term. When it comes to Weight Watchers, you are able to maintain it because it is so easy and simple to follow. You can live life while on this diet, still having a few treats and getting to eat out when you would like, but you just have to be a bit smarter about the choices that you make when it comes to the foods that you eat.

The Weight Watchers program is based on a points system. When you attend our first meeting or sign up online, you will be able to learn how many points you are allowed to have during the day. The points that you get will vary based on how much you want to lose, and some other factors including weight, age, height, and activity level. The point levels will change during your journey to help you adjust to any weight loss that you have and ensures that you will continue to see results along the way.

These points are going to really help you along the way. They don't tell you exactly what you have to eat, but they will help you to pick the right choices. Foods that are high in protein and lots of good nutrients, such as vegetables, fruits, and lean meats, will be lower in points. This means that you would be able to eat more of them before you met your point values. Options that are high in bad fats, carbs, and sugars are going to be higher in points. This means that you would be able to eat fewer of them before reaching your point allowance.

Now, you are able to have a treat on occasion if you would like, but you just need to be smart about how you are doing with it. Plus, if you are allowed to have a lot of one type of food when you are hungry and not so much of another, you are probably more likely to pick the food that is healthier so that you can eat a little bit more.

You can even use these points when you go out to eat. You will be able to learn how to calculate the points for what you would like to eat when you go out (and since the Weight Watchers plan is so prevalent, many restaurants will include the points totals for you on the menu), and then you can make smart choices that will help you to keep losing the weight, even when you want to go out and have some fun.

The idea behind the Weight Watchers plan is to not deprive you, but to just help you to make some healthier choices. This diet plan realizes that there are days when things are tough and you would like to eat something that is a little sweet or bad for you. It understands that there are times you want to go out and celebrate with friends and have some fun. There are no rules against doing these things you just need to learn how to use your points correctly so that you can really see the results.

In addition to being able to use the SmartPoints® to stay on track with your weight loss, you will find that the meetings are also helpful. These are available in many areas around the country, but if you aren't able to make the meeting times in your area or you are too far away from one, you can also do the meetings online. This is where you will meet others who are on the same journey as you, ask some of the questions that you have, get lots of advice, and even do your weigh-ins to see how you are doing. Don't worry about having to share your weight with anyone else. First this is a supportive community of people who are on the same journey as you are and second, you will be able to do the weigh-ins in private so you won't have to worry about anyone else knowing how well you are doing or if you fell behind on a week.

It is a really good idea to go to the meetings as often as you can. These help to hold you accountable and result in people on this plan losing a lot more weight than if they did it all on their own without the meetings. You are also going to meet a lot of amazing people who are trying to lose weight as well, or who already lost weight with this program, and they can give you inspiration to keep on working hard for the results that you want.

You should also make sure that you are getting in plenty of exercise during the week. This is a part that a lot of people miss out on sometimes, but it is so important for the overall health of your heart and body. While Weight Watchers has made some changes in terms of the relationship between their points and exercise in order to foster a healthier relationship between the two, it is still important to get some movement in each day to make the muscles and heart stronger. Try to do a combination of aerobics, weight lifting, and stretching on most days of the week to really help out with our weight loss goals.

There are also many health benefits that you can enjoy when using the Weight Watchers system. You will first notice that it helps you to lose a lot of weight. Since you are reducing a lot of the calories that you consume each day, you will be able to enjoy a lot of weight loss. Plus, your body is getting in so many good nutrients that it will feel like it is filled up and more energized than you did on your old diet plan.

You may also notice that your heart health is getting better than before. The healthy foods that you are eating, and the ones that you get rid of, will help to nourish the heart, limit high blood pressure, and can even take care of some of that cholesterol that is causing some issues. You may also notice that while you are on the Weight Watchers plan, you are eating fewer sugars so it is easier to lower your bad blood sugars and maybe even take care of some of those issues that come with diabetes.

Other benefits that you may notice while being on this simple diet plan includes more energy, better mood because your mind feels like it is opened up and ready to take on the day, lower joint pain from all that acidic food you are eating and so much more. There is just so much that you will be able to see improved when you are on the Weight Watchers plan that it is worth your time to give this diet plan a try.

If you are looking for a new diet plan and you are tired of all the hard work and impossible tasks that are placed out in some of your other diet plans of the past, it may be time to try out the Weight Watchers diet plan. This one is simple to use and will be able to help you get the results that you want without being impossible. While other diet plans have you eat things that are unhealthy or limit you so much that you are bound to fail at some point, Weight Watchers is meant for your daily life.

This diet plan allows you to have some of the snacks and some of the sweets that you crave, as long as you are careful about how you eat for the majority of the time. This diet realizes that you may have tough days or those days that you want to go out and celebrate, and it makes sure that you are getting the right nutrition while still eating out and having fun on occasion.

It also provides you with a support group to get through the good and the tough times when they come up. There is just so much to love about this particular diet plan and you are going to love how easy it is to get on and follow!

Why Choose Weight Watchers?

There are a lot of great diet plans that you can choose to go with. Some are going to choose to have you limit your carb intake while others are going to limit the fats. Some are healthy while others are going to be hard to maintain because they are so hard on the body. Weight Watchers is a bit different than all of these because you get some options. Some of the reasons that you should choose to go with Weight Watchers instead of another weight loss program includes:

- Lose more weight—overall, people who go on a program similar to Weight Watchers are able to lose more weight than with other options. This is because it is flexible to follow and you have that motivation and support going to the meetings each week.
- Flexibility—there is a lot of flexibility that comes with being on Weight Watchers. You get to enjoy the ability to pick the foods that you want to consume, when you want to eat them, and even how much based on the amount of points that you are going with. You can also pick your activity levels, your meetings, whether to have the meetings in person or online and so much more! This makes it easier for everyone to find the path on this plan that works best for them.
- Lifestyle change—weight watchers is not just about losing weight. It is about making changes in your whole lifestyle that will result in healthy weight loss. You are going to learn how to eat foods that are healthier and full of nutrition while getting rid of the foods that are causing weight gain and health issues. You are going to learn how important activity is in your life and star to implement it in more. You will work on getting healthier stress levels and sleeping as well.
- Eat the foods you like—you are the one in charge of the foods that you eat on this diet plan, so you can eat some of your favorites as well. While you do need to make some

healthier choices when it comes to staying within your points, there is still the option of having some of your favorite meals on occasion.
- Ability to fit it into your daily life—it is possible to fit this diet plan into your daily life. You are able to eat real foods, foods that taste good, and will fill you up. You can choose to workout each day or do normal activities, such as chores, around the house, without having to spend hours at the gym each day. The foods can be your normal favorites as long as you are careful about not eating too much.
- You can eat out—when you are on this plan, you are allowed to eat out. While you shouldn't do this each day, eating out every once in a while is not a bit sin of this diet plan. It realizes that there are times you will go out with friends and family and realizing that you can go out as long as you make the right decisions for the rest of the day and don't overdo it with eating at the restaurant, you will be fine without ruining all your hard work.
- People to help you along the way—there are weekly meetings that you can attend that will help you to stay on your plan. You can meet with others who will motivate you along your journey and will help you any time that things get stuff or you need some help. It is hard to find this kind of motivation on the other diet plans that you pick.

There is no diet plan that is the same as Weight Watchers for all the flexibility and support that you are going to get along the way. If you have been trying to lose weight in the past and are ready to take that step to seeing a lot of success finally, make sure to check out Weight Watchers and see how it can work for you.

What Foods Can I Eat?

One of the first questions that people are going to have when they get on the Weight Watchers program is what foods they are allowed to eat. You want to have a good idea of the foods that are allowed and the ones that aren't allowed so that you can plan accordingly when making your meals or going to the grocery store. When it comes to the Weight Watchers plan, you will see that you are not really limited on the types of food that you are allowed to eat, although you are certainly going to be guided to pick ones that are healthier. Weight Watchers understands that staying on a diet can be tough and if you are always told that you can't have something or you will lose all that hard work, you are going to crave that thing all the more. While you should concentrate on eating mostly healthy foods and staying in your allotted points, there is some freedom to have something a little "bad" for you on occasion and this is even added into the points that you can have each week.

This is not an invitation to eat as many of the bad things that you want each week and still hope to lose weight. There are a few extra points that are added to your weekly total, but they are not enough for you to go crazy with. They are there to allow you to get the amount of calories that you need to stay healthy and for a little bit of treat when you just can't fight the cravings.

While there aren't really any limits on the foods that you are able to eat, you do need to stick with the points that are given to you at the meeting. Keep in mind that as you lose weight these point amounts are going to go down a bit so that you are able to keep on losing weight. The beauty of these points is that they are going to help you to make the healthy choices, so you end up eating fewer calories, as well as better foods, in the long run.

Think of it this way, would you like to waste all of those points that you have for the day on a big coffee at Starbucks, or would it be better to have three nice meals with a lean protein, some milk, and some vegetables along with a nice snack of fruits? In most cases, you are going to go for the latter option because it helps you to feel full, gives your body the right nutrition, and can make you feel better. Of course, you are allowed to have that dessert on occasion, but you will learn that it isn't always worth it to give into the cravings and will instead pick to go with the healthier foods.

Started with Weight Watchers

It is actually pretty simple to get started with Weight Watchers. You will start out by finding a meeting that is in your area; if you find that the meetings are not in your area or you just aren't able to make the times that are in your area, you can also sign up for the meetings online as well. Even if you do want to go to the meetings in person most of the time, you may find that there are some great online tools that you are able to use to help you stay on track in between some of your meetings.

When you find a local Weight Watchers meeting, you are going to find that you are getting into a group that has a lot of great individuals. All of these people have either gone on their weight loss journey or are working on it at that time and all of them are on the Weight Watchers program. This can make it easier to connect to the people who are working towards the same goals as you and they will help you to stay on track, live a healthier lifestyle, and get the results that you want.

Some people are scared about doing these meetings, but there is nothing to worry about. They are a lot of fun, you get to meet new people and share stories, you get the encouragement that you need to feel amazing, and all of your results are going to be private so no one else will know!

Overall, this is one of the best diet plans that most people will choose to go with. it allows you to eat a lot of the foods that you enjoy while getting a few of those cheat days on occasion without having to worry about it all the time. While it will take some adjusting to look at the foods that you are eating based on how many points they are worth, the Weight Watchers plan can make it easier than ever to eat right, pick the foods that are healthier, and lose that weight, while gaining that good health, that you have been looking for.

Following Weight Watchers is a great option that is going to help you to not only lose weight, but also to take care of the other unhealthy parts of your diet. You are going to love not only that the inches are coming off, but that you are able to get more energy, that you feel better, and that your lifestyle in general is just better than before.

As this chapter and the rest of the guidebook talks about, Weight Watchers is a lifestyle change, one that you are able to maintain for the long term without having to starve yourself or feel miserable all the time. With the help of the points and meetings, you will find that Weight Watchers is not a fad and that you can make it work for you!

What are the SmartPoints®

With Weight Watchers, you are not necessarily kicking out any of the food groups, you are just becoming more conscious about the food decisions that you make.

This diet plan realizes that you are going to want that piece of cake or that cookies on occasion and telling you that you are not allowed to have it will simply make the situation worse. The idea behind Weight Watchers is that you are allowed to have some of these snacks and goodies, as long as you fit it properly within your diet.

When you go on Weight Watchers, you are going to be given a points system. This is to help you to make decisions based on your current weight and how much you would like to use in the process. These are the amount of points that you are able to use up during the day and can help you to make healthier food choices. Each food that you pick will have a certain point value and the goal is to stay within the points each day.

Now as mentioned, you are allowed to eat some of those sweets, but if you are at the end of the day and have only five points left, you may reach for an apple rather than going for that piece of cake that is worth 15 and would put you over your point goal.

You get to decide how to use the points and there are lots of handbooks that will help you to see how many points each of your food choices are. If you do want that piece of cake in the day (perhaps you know you are heading to a birthday party), you will be able to budget ahead of time to pick out wholesome and healthy foods that will keep you within your points allowance without missing out on nutrition.

You will need to be careful about these points. Some people get too excited about losing weight and will try to limit their calories too much. This may seem like a good idea; they assume that if they only use half their calories each day, they will lose the weight faster. But the issue here is that you may be cutting calories, but you are also cutting out healthy nutrition that the body really needs. You need to be careful about doing this.

There may be days when you aren't as hungry or you are too busy to eat as much as you should and your points values will be a bit lower. You don't need to force yourself to eat on these days. But you should aim to get close to your point totals each day so that you are giving your body adequate nutrition and calories to keep functioning.

These points are going to be really important when it comes to the foods that you are allowed to eat on this diet plan. Rather than focusing on the calories that you are consuming, you are going to focus on the points. These points are based on the macro and micro nutrients that are inside of the food that you plan to eat during the day.

When the food has a lot of good macro and micro nutrients like protein, good carbs, and healthy vitamins, you are going to see that they contain a smaller amount of points and you are able to eat more of them throughout the day with your diet.

On the other hand, if the items are mostly calories, sugars, and saturated fats, they are going to rank higher when it comes to the points that you are able to use. The idea behind this is that you are encouraged to eat more of the healthier foods while ditching some of the bad foods, although some of these bad foods are allowed on occasion when you are on the diet plan.

These points are going to allow you to make the best decisions when it is time to pick out the foods that you want to enjoy. You are going to be able to enjoy some of the treats on occasion when you want, but overall, you will choose to go out and eat the healthier foods because they fill you up more, you can eat more of them without having to use up all of your points, and they will taste so amazing in the process!

The Smart Points History

During 2016, Weight Watchers made some changes to their points system. They had received some criticism that their program was too much about the points and not enough about the nutritional content of the foods people were picking.

People could easily miss out on the healthy nutrients that they needed or pick foods that were high in sugars and saturated fats and still stick within the guidelines that were set out with Weight Watchers. This is why Weight Watchers came out with the new "Smart Points" and the "Beyond the Scale" program in 2016.

The Smart Points have made it easier to count out your points and they are going to push you towards foods that are healthier and more nutritious. This has a lot of great benefits including helping you to feel better, lose weight, and gain more energy at the same time. The food items that may have had lower points totals before, such as those with sugar and saturated fats, now have higher point values. Protein sources and fresh produce will have lower points values.

You are still in charge of the foods that you would like to eat, but the points are going to encourage you to pick foods that are healthier so that you are able to stay within your points value. The new point system is going to reward you for eating less saturated fat and less sugar while eating more protein in your diet.

The Activity Points have now been replaced with the FitPoints within Weight Watchers and they are going to be calculated out based on the activities that you are doing each week. The activities can range from planned exercises to just doing chores around the house during the day.

In addition to your normal points values that you are given, the original points in Weight Watchers would give you an extra 49 that you are able to use in the way that you wanted. These can be nice for that one cheat day or when you are just feeling really hungry on one of your days. The Smart Points still have these extra calories, but they are going to be adjusted based on the individual person and may include factors like age, gender, your goals for weight loss, and even your activity levels.

The benefits of the Smart Points

There are a lot of benefits that come from using Smart Points for your weight loss goals and this is part of why the Weight Watchers system is so popular. Some of the benefits of going with this system includes:

- The Smart Points help to keep you to pick healthier foods that are good for you. You will be docked any time that you choose foods that are full of sugars and saturated fats while

those who chose healthier options would be set.
- The Smart Points got rid of the unhealthy notion that if you exercise more, you can eat more. Most people overestimate their activity level so this led to them having issues with weight loss, plus they were still eating the unhealthy foods in the process. With the Smart Points, you will not be able to add in more points when you exercise more, so you will separate out the activity that you do from the foods that you eat.
- These Smart Points are going to focus more on having a healthier lifestyle. While weight loss is a part of this, you are going to find that it is more about the healthier lifestyle rather than just counting calories and worrying yourself sick over everything that you eat.

The negatives of Smart Points

While there are a lot of positives that you will be able to get from using the points system from Weight Watchers, there are a few people who have voiced concerns over the new Smart Points, especially those who were used to the old system with Weight Watchers. Some of the complaints that have come up in regards to these points include:

- Some people are worried that these points are making it more difficult to pick out foods. There isn't as much flexibility and freedom in the points. If you were used to the old Points Plus system, you may really notice this.
- There are a lot of restrictions. The restrictions for eating things like cake and cookies on the new Smart Points program is so high, that many will want to give up on the whole program. While it is an adjustment, most people who seriously

wanting to lose weight will not see an issue with these and will stay on the plan.

When you join Weight Watchers, you will be able to work with a coach, whether you work online or you go in person to the meetings. They will be able to fill out your profile to figure out how much you weight, how much you want to lose, how tall you are, your age, and other things that will influence your health and how much weight you can loose on the system. Things like being older in age or wanting to lose more weight will really slow down the metabolism and will need to be taken into consideration.

With this information, your coach will be able to determine how many points are a good place for you to start and will give you suggestions on staying healthy and making the right meal choices. Over time, you will be able to meet with your coach again and adjust the values based on whether you need to lose more weight, are losing too much weight, or just want to maintain the weight loss that you have already accomplished.

Either way, the points value system in Weight Watchers is a great way to get started on the system and will ensure that you are picking out the best foods for your body to stay healthy, get more energy, and to even lose some weight in the process. Keep in mind that when you get started on this whole program, you will lose weight in most cases, but the process is more about changing out the unhealthy aspects of your lifestyle rather than losing the weight.

Most of the other programs that you are going to choose will not work on this points system. They are going to just tell you the foods that you are allowed to eat and the ones that you should avoid. They will tell you how many calories that you should have and will place so many restrictions on you that it is too hard to keep up with during the daily life that you are living.

On the other hand, when you are using the SmartPoints® system, you aren't going to be so limited. You are able to take care of your own decisions when picking out foods. You can mix things up a bit and have a wide variety of foods rather than being stuck with just a few meals that fit in with the diet plan. When you are ready to try out something that is going to help you to lose weight while still maintaining some of your own individuality and without ruining your whole day, Weight Watchers is the best option for your weight loss goals.

There are some people who like using the SmartPoints® to help them to limit the bad foods and eat the good foods that will actually help them to lose the weight that they want. Others feel like this is too easy for some people and that it isn't really helping them to concentrate on the right foods in the right way since you are still allowed to eat some of the foods that are bad for you. Either way, this is one of the most popular diet plans on the market or many people have seen a lot of results when it comes to their health and weight loss goals with Weight Watchers.

WEIGHT WATCHERS FREESTYLE 2018

In November 2017, changes began to roll out and a new name was given to the plan. Instead of Beyond the Scale, it is now the **Flex Plan** in the UK and the **Freestyle Plan** in the US. Food points are still calculated using the same measurements of calories, fats, carbohydrates, and sugars. The biggest differences in the plan are listed below.

What's New Adding To The Program:

- **There are more free/zero point foods!** On the previous plan, most fruits and vegetables were zero Smart Points (they still are!) but now Weight Watchers has added a whole bunch of new foods to the "free" list. These foods don't need to be tracked or measured. Here's what is zero Smart Points on the new Freestyle plan:
    - **Fresh and frozen fruit** without added sugar, and canned fruits in water or sugar-free syrup (this has not changed)
    - **Most fresh and frozen vegetables** and those canned without oil or added sugar (this has not changed – excludes some vegetables such as potatoes, sweet potatoes, avocados, olives)
    - **Peas** – NEW! (includes chickpeas, sugar snap, snow, split, black-eyed)
    - **Beans** – NEW! (includes black, kidney, edamame, fat free refried, pinto, bean sprouts, soy beans)
    - **Lentils** – NEW!
    - **Corn** – NEW! (includes sweet corn, corn on the cob, baby corn)
    - **Skinless Chicken Breast** – NEW! (includes whole or ground chicken breast – if ground make sure it is breast meat only/98% fat free or higher)
    - **Skinless Turkey Breast** – NEW! (includes whole or ground turkey breast – if ground make sure it is breast meat only/98% fat free or higher)
    - **Tofu** – NEW!
    - **Eggs and Egg Whites** – NEW!

- **Nonfat Plain Yogurt** – NEW! (includes traditional, Greek, Icelandic, Soy)
- **Fish and Shellfish, skinless** – NEW! (includes fresh, frozen, canned, and smoked without added fat or sugar)

- **Your daily Smart Points allowance will change.** To balance out all the new zero point foods, your daily points will be recalculated (still according you your age, height, weight and gender). It appears to me that many members who were at 30 daily points on the previous plan will now be given 23 Smart Points per day on the Freestyle plan, but that may not be the case for everyone. If you're a current member, your daily points will be recalculated this week on your weigh in day.

- **Introducing Rollover Points!** On the Freestyle plan, you can roll over up to four unused daily points into your weekly points allowance to be used as extras whenever you like for the remainder of the week. For example, if you know you have a big event coming up later in the week, you can bank up to 4 unused points per day in the days leading up to it to make sure you have plenty of points to indulge at your event. To make use of this you'll want to be sure you're filling up on plenty of zero point foods on the days you're banking extra points.

WHAT'S STILL STAY:

- **Smart Points** – The new Weight Watchers Freestyle program still uses Smart Points with the same calculation, so the majority of foods (with the exception of the new zero point items) will keep the same Smart Points. Smart Points are calculated based on calories, saturated fat, sugar and protein. Saturated fat and sugar will increase a food's SP value while protein will lower the SP value.

- **Weekly Points Allowance** – while your daily points allowance will recalculate to make room for the new zero point foods, your weekly points will not differ based on the program changes.

How will this affect the existing Smart Points recipes?

Since the points on the new Freestyle plan will still be called Smart Points, but will be changing for many of new recipes, I will be labeling the updated points values as "Freestyle Smart Points." That way you should be able to easily designate which recipes have been updated and which I am still working on. I will try to get to everything as quickly as I can! Obviously a lot of my recipes include chicken breast, eggs, beans, corn, etc. so it likely won't be overnight. Thanks in advance for your patience, I will update this post with my progress.

As I've mentioned in the past, the Weight Watchers recipe builder does not count points for zero point foods. Because of this, the Smart Points you calculate using the recipe builder will not always match the Smart Points you get by entering the nutrition information for a recipe into the points calculator. Zero point foods still have calories, carbs, sugar, saturated fat, etc. and the nutrition information will reflect this! For this reason, I recommend using the recipe builder to calculate the SPs for recipes.

What do I think about the new Weight Watchers Freestyle Program?

Overall, I think this change could actually provide increased flexibility as long as you prepare and include the healthy zero point foods in your meal planning. To me this plan seems kind of like a blend of the previous Beyond the Scale Smart Points program and the Simply Filling plan (where you didn't have to track "power foods"). It certainly leads you to incorporate healthy, lean (zero point) foods into your diet. Here are some of my thoughts in no particular order:

- **Easier for Vegetarians** – the fact that eggs, beans, tofu, lentils, plain FF yogurt, etc. are all zero points means vegetarians following the Freestyle plan have a lot more flexibility and more filling, low point options/protein sources.
- **Planning/Food Prep/Grocery Shopping is Key** – making a batch of my Easy Slow Cooker Shredded Chicken, for example, can really set you up for success for the week! Make sure to stock up on the new zero point foods to get the most bang for your buck on the new plan. Since your daily points allowance will be lower, the Freestyle plan will be tough if you are not incorporating some of the new zero point foods.
- **Ground Chicken/Turkey Breast vs Ground Beef** – I know a lot of you will want to make my ground beef recipes with ground chicken breast or turkey breast now that they are free. I love lean ground beef and am still going to keep using it in recipes, but I will try to also provide an alternate Smart Points calculation for making the recipe with a zero point meat option. At first when I saw the new plan I worried that no one would eat beef anymore, but then I realized the flexibility of the new program leaves plenty of room for steak or ground beef. If I have eggs and yogurt and fruit for breakfast and chicken with veggies for lunch I could eat a *giant* portion of steak for dinner and still have points for dessert!
- **Easier to Plan for Indulgences** – not only do you have the same weekly points to use to plan for a few glasses of wine, a dessert or a special event, but you can now easily bulk up on filling zero point foods to save your dailies and even roll over unused dailies to use later in the week. This is great for planning a night out with friends, a weekend away,

a holiday splurge, or whatever you most enjoy. You can also plan for daily indulgences (like full fat cheese or snack foods) fairly easily so long as you incorporate some of the healthy zero point foods into your day.

- **Some Fun New Free Options** – though I will always wish avocado would be free, I'm excited to see beans (including fat free refried which I love as a side dish), corn, chickpeas, nonfat plain yogurt, corn, edamame, eggs and chicken breast. I love all those things! I wish I was a seafood lover, but sadly it is not for me. It'll be great for those of you who are though!

Some of additions to the Zero Points Food List:

Black beans, Great Northern Beans, Kidney Beans, and Pinto Beans

Tofu, Smoked Tofu, and some other meat substitutes

Chicken breast, turkey breast, and some brands of sugar-free chicken or turkey luncheon meats

Eggs (both whole and egg whites)

Nonfat Unsweetened Yogurt

Corn and peas of many kinds

Fish and Shellfish (including canned tuna in water)

For more information about the program if you're a member, check in with your Weight Watchers leader or on the Weight Watchers website. You can always use their 24/7 chat if you're a member who has questions.

So here they are some of my latest Freestyle SmartPoints Recipes.

FREESTYLE SMARTPOINTS RECIPES

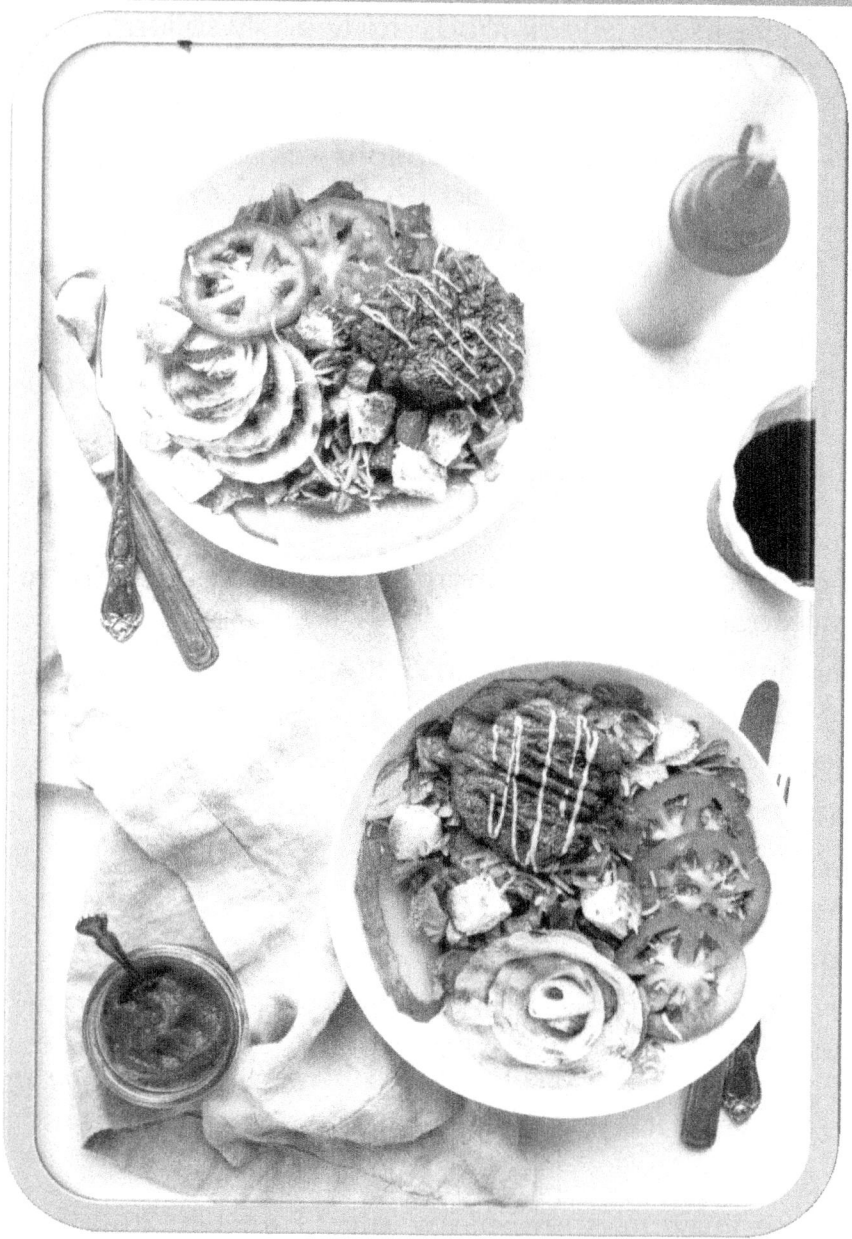

FREESTYLE BUTTER CHICKEN POT PASTA

Yield: 8 (1 1/4 CUPS) SERVINGS

INGREDIENTS:
- 1 ½ lbs. uncooked boneless, skinless chicken breasts
- 4 tablespoons light butter
- ½ cup chopped onion
- ¼ cup flour
- ½ teaspoon salt
- ¼ teaspoon black pepper
- 1 ½ cups skim milk
- 2 ½ cups water*
- 1 tablespoon Better Than Bouillon Roasted Chicken Base
- ½ teaspoon poultry seasoning
- 8 oz. uncooked egg noodles
- 1 cup frozen corn kernels
- 2 cups frozen peas and carrots

DIRECTIONS:
1. Place the chicken breasts in a Dutch oven or other large pot and cover with water to about 2 inches over the chicken.
2. Bring the water to a boil over high heat and then reduce the heat to medium. Cook over medium heat for 15-20 minutes (depending on the thickness of your chicken breasts – mine are generally done at 15, so check one then) until chicken is cooked through.
3. Remove the chicken breasts to a cutting board. Discard the water from the pot and rinse and wipe out the pot to use again. Chop the chicken into small, bite-size pieces and set aside.

4. Melt the butter in the pot over medium heat. Add the chopped onion and cook for a few minutes until the onion is softened.
5. Whisk in the flour, salt and pepper until combined with the butter and onions and continue to whisk for another 1-2 minutes.
6. Slowly whisk in the milk until combined and smooth. Add the water and bouillon base (or broth) and poultry seasoning and whisk in to combine.
7. Increase the heat to med-high and stir occasionally until boiling. Reduce the heat to med-low and add the egg noodles. Cook for 8 minutes, stirring regularly to prevent sticking. If you need a little more liquid toward the end you can add a bit more water or broth.
8. Add the chopped chicken, corn, and peas and carrots and stir until thoroughly combined. Cook for another few minutes until all ingredients are heated through.

WEIGHT WATCHERS FREESTYLE SMARTPOINTS:
5 per (1 ¼ cup) serving (*SPs calculated using the recipe builder on weightwatchers.com*), a serving was 8 SPs on the previous program

WEIGHT WATCHERS POINTS PLUS:
8 per (1 ¼ cup) serving (*PP calculated using a WW PointsPlus calculator and the nutrition info below*)

NUTRITION INFORMATION PER (1 ¼ CUP) SERVING:
314 calories, 35 g carbs, 3 g sugars, 7 g fat, 2 g saturated fat, 27 g protein, 3 g fiber

FREESTYLE ONE POT GARLICKY CUBAN PORK

5 Smart Points 213 calories

TOTAL TIME: 80 minutes plus marinade time

INGREDIENTS:

- 3 lb. boneless pork shoulder blade roast, lean, all fat removed
- 6 cloves garlic
- juice of 1 grapefruit (about 2/3 cup)
- juice of 1 lime
- 1/2 tablespoon fresh oregano
- 1/2 tablespoon cumin
- 1 tablespoon kosher salt
- 1 bay leaf
- lime wedges, for serving
- chopped cilantro, for serving
- hot sauce, for serving
- tortillas, optional for serving
- salsa, optional for serving

DIRECTIONS:

1. PRESSURE COOKER: Cut the pork in 4 pieces and place in a bowl.
2. In a small blender or mini food processor, combine garlic, grapefruit juice, lime juice, oregano, cumin and salt and blend until smooth.
3. Pour the marinade over the pork and let it sit room temperature 1 hour or refrigerated as long as overnight.

4. Transfer to the pressure cooker, add the bay leaf, cover and cook high pressure 80 minutes. Let the pressure release naturally.
5. Remove pork and shred using two forks.
6. Remove liquid from pressure cooker, reserving then place the pork back into pressure cooker. Add about 1 cup of the liquid (jus) back, adjust the salt as needed and keep warm until you're ready to eat.

1. SLOW COOKER: Cut the pork in 4 pieces and place in a bowl.
2. In a small blender or mini food processor, combine garlic, grapefruit juice, lime juice, oregano, cumin and salt and blend until smooth.
3. Pour the marinade over the pork and let it sit room temperature 1 hour or refrigerated as long as overnight.
4. Transfer to the slow cooker, add the bay leaf, cover and cook low 8 hours.
5. Remove pork and shred using two forks.
6. Remove liquid from slow cooker, reserving then place the pork back into slow cooker. Add about 1 cup of the liquid (jus) back, adjust the salt as needed and keep warm until you're ready to eat.

NUTRITION INFORMATION
Yield: 10 servings, Serving Size: a little over 3 oz.
Amount Per Serving:
Smart Points: 5, Points +: 5, Calories: 213, Total Fat: 9.5g
Saturated Fat: 0g, Cholesterol: 91mg, Sodium: 440.5mg
Carbohydrates: 2.5g, Fiber: 0.5g, Sugar: 1.5g
Protein: 26.5g

FREESTYLE PIMENTO CHILE CHICKEN

Ingredients:
- 2 ½ c. cooked, chopped chicken breast (chopped into about 1/2" cubes
- ½ c. fat free chicken broth
- 1 ½ c. 98% fat free cream of mushroom soup (I use Campbell's)
- 1 ½ c. Healthy Request Condensed cream of chicken soup
- 1 4-oz. jar pimentos, drained (1/2 c.)
- 2 4-oz. cans Hatch green chiles, chopped and drained (You can add a 3rd can if you're just crazy about chiles like I am.)
- 10 oz. 50% reduced fat sharp cheddar cheese
- 6 oz. of Doritos (by weight) toasted corn tortilla chips, slightly crushed
- Pickled jalapeños, green onions, and/or cherry tomatoes for serving (optional)

Instructions:
1. Mix all ingredients except Doritos and cheese. In a large casserole dish (I use 9" x 13"), layer ½ of chicken mixture, then ½ of cheese, then ½ of the Doritos.
2. Repeat the same layers once more, ending with Doritos on top. Bake at 350° for about 40-45 minutes.
3. Cover top with foil if Doritos begin to brown too much. Serve with pickled jalapeños and/or your favorite salsa.

Weight Watchers Info: 6 points per serving in the new Freestyle plan; makes 8 servings.

FREESTYLE WHITE CHICKEN CHILI

Yield: 8 (1 CUP) SERVINGS

INGREDIENTS:

- 1 tablespoon Canola oil
- 2 cups yellow onion, chopped
- 2 tablespoons chili powder
- 1 tablespoon minced garlic
- 2 teaspoons ground cumin
- 1 teaspoon oregano
- 3 (15.5 oz.) cans Great Northern beans, rinsed and drained
- 4 cups reduced sodium fat free chicken broth
- 3 cups chopped or shredded cooked skinless chicken breast
- 1 (14.5 oz.) can diced tomatoes
- 1/3 cup chopped fresh cilantro
- 2 tablespoon fresh lime juice
- ½ teaspoon salt
- ½ teaspoon pepper

DIRECTIONS:

1. Bring oil to medium heat in a large pot or Dutch oven. Add the onions and sauté for 5-8 minutes or until tender.
2. Add the chili powder, garlic and cumin and stir to coat the onions. Cook for 2 more minutes. Add the oregano and beans, stir and cook for 30 more seconds.
3. Add the broth and reduce the heat to medium-low. Simmer for 20 minutes, stirring occasionally.

4. Remove 2 cups of the bean/broth mixture into a blender (or container for an immersion blender) and process until smooth.
5. Return pureed mixture to the pot. Add the chicken and tomatoes and cook over medium-low for another 30 minutes, stirring occasionally.
6. Add the cilantro, lime juice, salt & pepper and stir to combine before serving.

WEIGHT WATCHERS FREESTYLE SMARTPOINTS:
1 per (1 cup) serving (SP *calculated using the recipe builder on weightwatchers.com*), a serving was 7 SPs on the previous program

WEIGHT WATCHERS POINTS PLUS:
7 per (1 cup) serving (P+ *calculated using the recipe builder on weightwatchers.com*)

NUTRITION INFORMATION PER 1 CUP SERVING:
291 calories, 36 g carbs, 4 g sugars, 4 g fat, 1 g saturated fat, 27 g protein, 12 g fiber

FREESTYLE BUFFALO WING HUMMUS

Yield: 8 (1/4 CUP) SERVINGS

INGREDIENTS:

- 1 ½ cups canned chickpeas, drained and rinsed (reserve ¼ cup of the liquid from the can)
- 2 cloves garlic
- 2 tablespoons tahini
- 2 tablespoons fresh lemon juice
- ¾ teaspoon paprika
- 1 tablespoon barbecue sauce
- 1 ½ tablespoons Frank's Red Hot (or similar cayenne pepper sauce)
- 1 ½ teaspoons white vinegar
- ¾ teaspoon salt

DIRECTIONS:

1. Combine all ingredients including the ¼ reserved liquid from the can of chickpeas into a food processor or blender. Puree ingredients until smooth. Serve.

WEIGHT WATCHERS FREESTYLE SMARTPOINTS:
1 per serving (SP *calculated using the recipe builder on weightwatchers.com*), a serving was 2 SmartPoints on the previous program

WEIGHT WATCHERS POINTS PLUS:
2 per serving (P+ *calculated using the recipe builder on weightwatchers.com*)

NUTRITION INFORMATION:
72 calories, 12 g carbs, 1 g sugars, 2 g fat, 0 g saturated fat, 3 g protein, 2 g fiber

FREESTYLE HAM AND CHEESE EGG CUPS

Yield: 12 EGG CUPS

INGREDIENTS:

- 9 oz. thinly sliced deli ham, divided (I used Hillshire Farm Deli Select)
- 6 large eggs
- 2 egg whites
- ¼ cup skim milk
- ¼ teaspoon salt
- 1/8 teaspoon pepper
- ½ cup chopped fresh spinach leaves
- 2 oz. shredded 2% sharp cheddar cheese, divided

DIRECTIONS:

1. Preheat the oven to 350. Lightly mist 12 cups in a muffin tin with cooking spray. Press a slice of ham into each cup of the muffin tin, arranging the edges to form a ham cup.
2. Chop up the remaining ham (my slices were about ½ ounce each so I had around 3 ounces remaining) and set aside.
3. In a mixing bowl, combine the eggs, egg whites, milk, salt and pepper and whisk together until yolks and whites are fully combined and beaten.
4. Add the reserved chopped ham, the spinach and half of the shredded cheddar and stir together to combine.
5. Spoon the egg mixture evenly into the ham cups and then top each cup with the remaining shredded cheese. Place the tin in the oven and bake for 18-20 minutes until the eggs are set.

WEIGHT WATCHERS FREESTYLE SMARTPOINTS:
1 per egg cup (*SP calculated using the recipe builder on weightwatchers.com*)

WEIGHT WATCHERS POINTS PLUS:
2 per egg cup (*P+ calculated using the recipe builder on weightwatchers.com*)

NUTRITION INFORMATION PER EGG CUP:
82 calories, 2 g carbs, 1 g sugars, 4 g fat, 2 g saturated fat, 9 g protein, 0 g fiber

FREESTYLE CORN AND ZUCCHINI SUMMER FRITTATA

Yield: 6 SLICES

INGREDIENTS:

- 1 medium ear of fresh raw corn
- 1 tablespoon light butter (I use Land O'Lakes)
- 1 cup thin sliced zucchini
- 8 large eggs
- 1/3 cup 2% plain Greek yogurt (I used Fage)
- ¾ teaspoon salt (plus a sprinkle more for the corn & zucchini)
- ¼ teaspoon black pepper (plus a sprinkle more for the corn & zucchini)
- 1 tablespoon diced chives
- ¼ cup sliced fresh basil
- 2 oz. sharp cheddar cheese, shredded (I used Cabot Seriously Sharp)

DIRECTIONS:

1. Pre-heat your oven to 350. Shuck the corn and remove any remaining strings. Use a large sharp knife to cut off the kernels as close to the cob as you can get (I ended up with about 1 cup of kernels).
2. Melt the butter in an 8"-10" *oven-safe* nonstick deep skillet over medium-low heat. Add the corn kernels and the sliced zucchini and stir to coat.
3. Sprinkle with a bit of salt and pepper to taste. Cook, stirring regularly, for 6-8 minutes or until corn and zucchini are cooked through.

4. While the corn and zucchini are cooking, break the eggs into a large mixing bowl and whisk together until just combined.
5. Add the yogurt, salt, black pepper, chives, basil and shredded cheese and stir together until mixed.
6. When the corn and zucchini are cooked, transfer them into the bowl containing the egg mixture and stir together. Spray the skillet you used liberally with cooking spray and then pour the egg mixture into the skillet.
7. Cook on a burner set to medium heat for 5-7 minutes until the very outside edge of the frittata starts to turn opaque/look cooked.
8. Transfer the skillet into the oven and cook for 15-17 minutes until the center is set. Let cool for 5 minutes, then slice into 6 slices and serve.

WEIGHT WATCHERS FREESTYLE SMARTPOINTS:
2 per slice (SP *calculated using the recipe builder on weightwatchers.com*), a serving was 5 SPs on the previous program

WEIGHT WATCHERS POINTS PLUS:
4 per slice (P+ *calculated using a Weight Watchers brand PointsPlus calculator and the nutrition information below*)

NUTRITION INFORMATION PER SLICE:
167 calories, 5 g carbs, 2 g sugars, 11 g fat, 5 g saturated fat, 13 g protein, 1 g fiber

TURKEY MEATBALL & VEGGIE SOUP

Nutrition Information
- Serves: 8 servings
- Serving size: 1-1/2 cup soup
- Calories: 285
- Fat: 13 g
- Saturated fat: 4 g
- Trans fat: 0 g
- Carbohydrates: 21 g
- Sugar: 9 g
- Sodium: 1126 mg
- Fiber: 3 g
- Protein: 19 g

Makes 8 servings.
One serving is 1-1/2 cups soup.
One serving is 5 FreeStyle WW SP.INGREDIENTS
- Cooking spray
- 1 onion, chopped
- 3-4 carrots, sliced or chopped
- 1 cup green beans, cut
- 2 minced garlic cloves
- 1 (24 ounce) package Jennie-O Italian style turkey meatballs
- 2 (14.5 ounce) cans beef or vegetable broth
- 2 (14.5 ounce) diced or Italian stewed tomatoes
- 1-1/2 cups frozen corn
- 1 teaspoon oregano
- 1 teaspoon parsley

- ½ teaspoon basil

INSTRUCTIONS

1. Spray large saucepan or instant pot with cooking spray.
2. Add onions, carrots, green beans and garlic and cook over medium heat 2-3 minutes.
3. Mix in remaining ingredients.
4. If cooking on a stovetop, cover and cook over medium-low heat for 20 minutes, or until meatballs are heated through.
5. -OR-
6. If using an instant pot, press the "soup" button and cook on high pressure for 15 minutes. Vent to release pressure once cooked.
7. -OR-
8. Cook in a slow cooker for 5-6 hours on LOW.
9. Serve warm.
10. Refrigerate or freeze leftovers.

FREESTYLE SHREDDED MEXICAN CHICKEN

Yield: 6 (1/2 CUP) SERVINGS

INGREDIENTS:

- 2 (8 oz.) cans tomato sauce
- 2 teaspoons white wine vinegar
- 3 cloves garlic, minced
- 4 teaspoons chili powder
- 1 teaspoon ground cumin
- 2 teaspoon oregano
- ½ teaspoon sugar
- Salt & pepper to taste
- 1 tablespoon extra virgin olive oil
- 1 small onion, chopped
- 1 ½ lbs. boneless, skinless chicken breasts

DIRECTIONS:

1. In a medium bowl, mix together the tomato sauce, vinegar, garlic, chili powder, cumin, oregano, sugar, salt and pepper until thoroughly combined.
2. In a large skillet or sauté pan, bring the oil to medium-high heat. Add the chopped onions and cook for a couple minutes until they start to soften and become fragrant.
3. Add the chicken breasts in a single layer and cook for 3 minutes on one side, flip them over, and then continue to cook for 3 minutes on the other side.
4. Add the tomato sauce mixture to the pan and bring it to a boil. Lower the heat to medium-low and cover the pan. Simmer for about 20 minutes until the chicken is fully cooked through.

5. Remove the lid from the pan and transfer each breast to a cutting board, shredding it using two forks and then returning it to the sauce.
6. When all the breasts are shredded, stir them into the sauce until thoroughly combined. Continue to cook for about 5 more minutes until the sauce thickens and soaks into the chicken.

WEIGHT WATCHERS FREESTYLE SMARTPOINTS:
1 per serving (SP *calculated using the recipe builder on weightwatchers.com*), a serving was 3 SmartPoints on the previous program

WEIGHT WATCHERS POINTS PLUS:
4 per serving (P+ *calculated using the recipe builder on weightwatchers.com*)

NUTRITION INFORMATION:
184 calories, 9 g carbs, 5 g sugars, 4 g fat, 1 g saturated fat, 26 g protein, 2 g fiber

FREESTYLE BAKED CHICKEN TENDERS

Yield: 4 (ROUGHLY 5.25 OUNCE) SERVINGS

INGREDIENTS:
- 4 teaspoons flour
- ½ teaspoon paprika
- 1.25 lbs. raw boneless skinless chicken breast tenderloins (you can also buy breasts and cut them into strips)
- 2 egg whites, beaten
- ½ cup cornflake crumbs (these are sold by the other bread crumbs in my stores, no need to crush your own!)
- ½ teaspoon dried parsley flakes
- ½ teaspoon salt
- ¼ teaspoon black pepper
- ¼ teaspoon cayenne pepper
- ¼ teaspoon onion powder
- ¼ teaspoon garlic powder

DIRECTIONS:
1. Pre-heat the oven to 375 degrees. Line a baking sheet with parchment paper and set aside.
2. In a small dish, mix together the flour and paprika. Place the chicken strips into a gallon Ziploc bag and add the flour/paprika mixture. Seal the bag and shake to coat the chicken.
3. In a shallow dish, beat the egg whites and set aside. In a separate shallow dish, stir together the cornflake crumbs, parsley, salt, pepper, cayenne, onion powder and garlic powder.
4. One at a time, take the flour-coated chicken strips and coat them in the egg whites and then press

them into the dish of corn flake crumbs and flip so that both sides are coated in crumbs.
5. Transfer the crumb-coated strips to the prepared baking sheet.
6. When all the chicken tenders are coated and on the baking sheet, spray the tops of them with cooking spray and place in the oven to bake for 18-20 minutes until cooked through.

WEIGHT WATCHERS FREESTYLE SMARTPOINTS:
2 per serving* (*SP calculated using the recipe builder on weightwatchers.com*), a serving was 4 SPs on the previous program

WEIGHT WATCHERS POINTS PLUS:
6 per serving* (*PP calculated using a Weight Watchers PointsPlus calculator and the nutrition information below*)

NUTRITION INFORMATION PER SERVING*:
229 calories, 12 g carbs, 1 g sugar, 4 g fat, 1 g saturated fat, 35 g protein, 0 g fiber

FREESTYLE THE BEST TURKEY CHILI

Yield: 12 (1-1/4 CUP) SERVINGS

INGREDIENTS:
- 2 tablespoons olive oil
- 2 cups diced onions (about 3 medium onions)
- 1 medium zucchini, diced
- 3 garlic cloves, minced
- 2 pounds 93% lean ground turkey
- 2 (28 oz.) cans diced tomatoes
- 1 (14 oz.) can Italian stewed whole tomatoes, roughly chopped
- 1 (6 oz.) can tomato paste
- 2 (15 oz.) cans cannellini beans, drained and rinsed (could also use kidney beans)
- 5 tablespoons chili powder
- 1 tablespoon cumin
- 1 teaspoon cayenne pepper
- 2 teaspoons salt
- 3 tablespoons chopped cilantro

DIRECTIONS:
1. Bring oil over medium heat in a large soup pot. Add the onion, zucchini and garlic and sauté for about 5 minutes until softened.
2. Add the ground turkey and continue to cook for another 6-7 minutes, stirring to cook evenly and breaking up the meat until the meat is cooked through.
3. Add the tomatoes, tomato paste, beans, chili powder, cumin, cayenne, salt and cilantro and stir to combine.

4. Reduce the heat and simmer uncovered for about an hour to thicken.

WEIGHT WATCHERS FREESTYLE SMARTPOINTS:
2 SP per serving if you use ground turkey breast
(SP *calculated using the recipe builder on weightwatchers.com*)

OR 6 per serving with the 93% lean ground turkey
(SP *calculated using the recipe builder on weightwatchers.com*)

WEIGHT WATCHERS POINTS PLUS:
6 per serving (P+ *calculated using the recipe builder on weightwatchers.com*)

NUTRITION INFORMATION:
278 calories, 28 g carbs, 9 g sugars, 8 g fat, 2 g saturated fat, 21 g protein, 7 g fiber

FREESTYLE MEXICAN CHICKEN CAULIFLOWER

Yield: 4 (1 CHICKEN + 1 CUP RICE MIX) SERVINGS

INGREDIENTS:

- 4 (4 oz.) thin chicken breast cutlets (I butterfly two 8 oz. breasts and then cut them to make two thin cutlets)
- 3 tablespoons taco seasoning, divided
- 1 tablespoon olive oil
- 12 oz. riced cauliflower (I used Green Giant frozen – no need to defrost)
- 1 cup salsa (I *highly* recommend using roasted tomato salsa – Wegmans, Frontera, Trader Joe's, etc. all have one)
- ¼ cup water
- ½ cup frozen corn kernels
- ¾ cup drained and rinsed canned black beans
- 2 oz. 50% reduced fat sharp cheddar cheese, shredded

DIRECTIONS:

1. Place the chicken breast cutlets in a gallon zip-top bag and add two tablespoons of the taco seasoning. Seal the bag and toss to coat the chicken in the seasoning.
2. In a large sauté pan or walled skillet, bring the olive oil over medium heat. Add the chicken in a single layer and cook on one side for 3-4 minutes.
3. Flip each piece and cook for an additional 3 minutes or until each piece is cooked through. Transfer the chicken to a side plate and cover with aluminum foil to keep warm.

4. Add the cauliflower rice, salsa, water, the remaining tablespoon of taco seasoning, corn and black beans to the skillet and stir to combine.
5. Cover and cook over medium for 5 minutes. Remove the lid to stir, cover and reduce heat to medium-low. Continue to cook for another 5 minutes or until the cauliflower is softened.
6. Remove the lid, stir the contents and then sprinkle the cheese over the top. Add the reserved chicken in a single layer on top of the cheese and replace the lid.
7. Turn off the burner and let the skillet sit, covered, for 1-2 minutes until the cheese is melted.

WEIGHT WATCHERS FREESTYLE SMARTPOINTS:
3 per (1 piece chicken + 1 cup "rice" mixture) serving (*SPs calculated using the recipe builder on weightwatchers.com*), a serving was 7 SPs on the previous plan

WEIGHT WATCHERS POINTS PLUS:
8 per (1 piece chicken + 1 cup "rice" mixture) serving (*PP calculated using a WW PointsPlus calculator and the nutrition info below*)

NUTRITION INFORMATION PER (1 PIECE CHICKEN + 1 CUP "RICE" MIXTURE) SERVING:
316 calories, 23 g carbs, 4 g sugars, 9 g fat, 3 g saturated fat, 35 g protein, 5 g fiber

ABILITY TO ROLL OVER DAILY POINTS TO YOUR WEEKLIES

Going back to an older plan favorite, you can now roll over up to 4 SmartPoints per day into your weekly points allowance. This makes it easier to splurge on a special treat and makes you feel less guilty about not eating all of your points each day.

The point is not to eat every single point, but to eat healthy foods until you are satiated. This promotes a healthier mindset and will help you to maintain good habits after you reach your goal.

Below are the 30 day meal plan that use the old smart points system which will still effective and get any one started the program easily.

A 30 DAY MEAL PLAN TO GET YOU STARTED

Sometimes one of the hardest things that you will need to do when it comes to getting started on a new meal plan is figure out what meals you would like to cook. There are so many meals out there, but learning which ones belong to your new diet plan and will not make you go over our daily limit can be kind of intimidating in the beginning.

In this chapter, we provide you with a 30-day meal plan that you can follow. There are lots of tasty recipes that you can try and you can find the recipes for all of them inside this guidebook. Whether you are looking for something light on the run or something that is a bit heartier for at night, you are sure to find many recipes that you can love on this list.

So try a few of them out, or use this as your meal planner, and get ready to find out just how great Weight Watchers can be and just how much weight you can lose.

| Day One: | Breakfast: Pancakes = 6
Lunch: Creamy Pesto Pasta = 7
Dinner: Spinach and Chicken Casserole = 4 |

	Total Points: 17 Points
Day Two:	Breakfast: Healthy Morning Cookies = 2 Lunch: BBQ Pork Sandwich = 5 Dinner: Vegetable Quesadilla = 9 Total Points: 16 Points
Day Three:	Breakfast: Cinnamon Rolls = 6 Lunch: Italian Chicken = 5 Dinner: Veggie Pork Chops = 6 Total Points: 17 Points
Day Four:	Breakfast Mushroom and Spinach Quchie = 3 Lunch: Baked Tortellini = 6 Dinner: Cheese Tuna Sandwich = 10 : Total Points: 19 Points
Day Five:	Breakfast: Apple Muffin: 7 Lunch: Cheesy Mushrooms = 2 Dinner: Cheeseburger Soup = 9 : Total Points:17 Points
Day Six	Breakfast: Potato and Cheese Casserole = 7 Lunch: Baked Burrito = 6 Dinner: Beef Chili = 3 : Total Points: 15 Points
Day Seven	Breakfast: Crispy Apple Surprise = 11 Lunch: Veggie Soup = 1 Dinner: Cilantro Lime Shrimp = 3 Total Points: 15 Points
Day Eight:	Breakfast: Breakfast Jelly Pudding = 11 Lunch: Veggie Soup = 1

	Dinner: Spinach and Chicken Crescents = 4 : Total Points:16 Points
Day Nine	Pumpkin Muffins = 4 Lunch: Italian Bread and Tuna Salad = 10 Dinner: Cheesy Chicken Cops = 3 : Total Points:17 Points
Day Ten:	Breakfast: Blackberry and Peach Smoothie = 9 Lunch: Cheeseburger Soup = 7 Dinner Cilantro Lime Shrimp = 3 : Total Points: 19 Points
Day eleven:	Breakfast: Morning Burritos = 9 Lunch: Pasta Veggies = 5 Dinner: Jalapeno Chicken = 4 : Total Points: 18 Points
Day Twelve	Breakfast Soufflé = 3 Lunch: Turkey and Cheese Sandwich = 10 Dinner: Jalapeno Chicken = 4 : Total Points: 17 Points
Day thirteen	Breakfast: Breakfast Bars = 6 Lunch: Creamy Pesto Pasta = 7 Dinner: Honey Salmon = 4 : Total Points:17 Points
Day Fourteen	Breakfast: French Toast = 3 Lunch: Baked Fish = 5 Dinner: Mexican Casserole = 8

	Total Points: 16 Points
Day fifteen:	Breakfast: Cheese and Ham Omelet = 6 Lunch: Beef Ziti Bake = 7 Dinner: Cheesy Chicken Chops = 3 Total Points:16 Points
Day sixteen:	Breakfast: Spiced Honey Cake = 7 Lunch: Chicken Salad = 4 Diner: Veggie Pork Chops = 6 Total Points: 17 Points
Day seventeen	Breakfast: Blueberry Muffins = 5 Lunch:: BBQ Pork Sandwich = 5 Dinner: Steak and Mashed Potatoes = 9 Total Points: 18 Pointes
Day eighteen	Breakfast: Yogurt Fluff = 2 Lunch: Baked Fish = 5 Dinner: Pita Bread Pizza =9 Total Points: 16 Points
Day nineteen	Breakfast: Pancakes = 6 Lunch: Bacon Wraps = 8 Dinner: Egg Salad = 4 Total Points: 19 Points
Day twenty	Breakfast: Healthy Morning Cookies = 2 Lunch: Beef Burgers = 4 Dinner: Roast Beef with Veggies = 9 Total Points: 14 Points
Day twenty-one	Breakfast: Cinnamon Rolls = 6 Lunch: Cheesy Mushrooms = 2

	Dinner: Cheese and Tuna Sandwich = 10 Total Points: 18 Points
Day twenty-two	Breakfast: Mushroom and Spinach Quiche = 3 Lunch: Beef Ziti Bake = 7 Dinner: Vegetable Quesadilla = 9 Total Points 19 Points
Day twenty-three	Breakfast: Apple Muffin = 7 Lunch: Chicken Salad = 4 Dinner: Chicken Thai Wrap = 2 Total Points: 13 Points
Day twenty-four	Breakfast: Potato and Cheese Casserole = 7 Lunch: Bacon wrap = 8 Dinner: Beef Chili = 2 Total Points: 19 Points
Day twenty-five	Breakfast: Pumpkin Muffins = 4 Lunch: Italian Bread with Tuna Salad = 10 Dinner: Cola Chicken = 5 Total Points 19 Points
Day twenty-six	Breakfast: Blackberry and Peach Smoothie = 9 Lunch: Beef Burgers = 4 Dinner: Mushroom Steak = 5 Total Points: 18 Points
Day twenty-seven	Breakfast: Morning Burritos = 9 Lunch: Pasta Veggies = 5 Dinner: Beef Chili = 2

	Total Points 18 Points
Day twenty0eght	Breakfast: Breakfast Soufflé = 3 Lunch: Baked Burrito = 6 Dinner: Baked Chicken = 10 : Total Points:19 Points
Day twenty-nine	Breakfast: Breakfast Bars = 6 Lunch: Baked Tortellini = 6 Dinner: Potato Soup = 4 Total Points: 18 Points
Day thirty	Breakfast: French Toast = 3 Lunch: Italian Chicken = 5 Dinner: Chicken Dumplings = 9 Total Points = 17 Points

WEIGHT WATCHERS BREAKFASTS

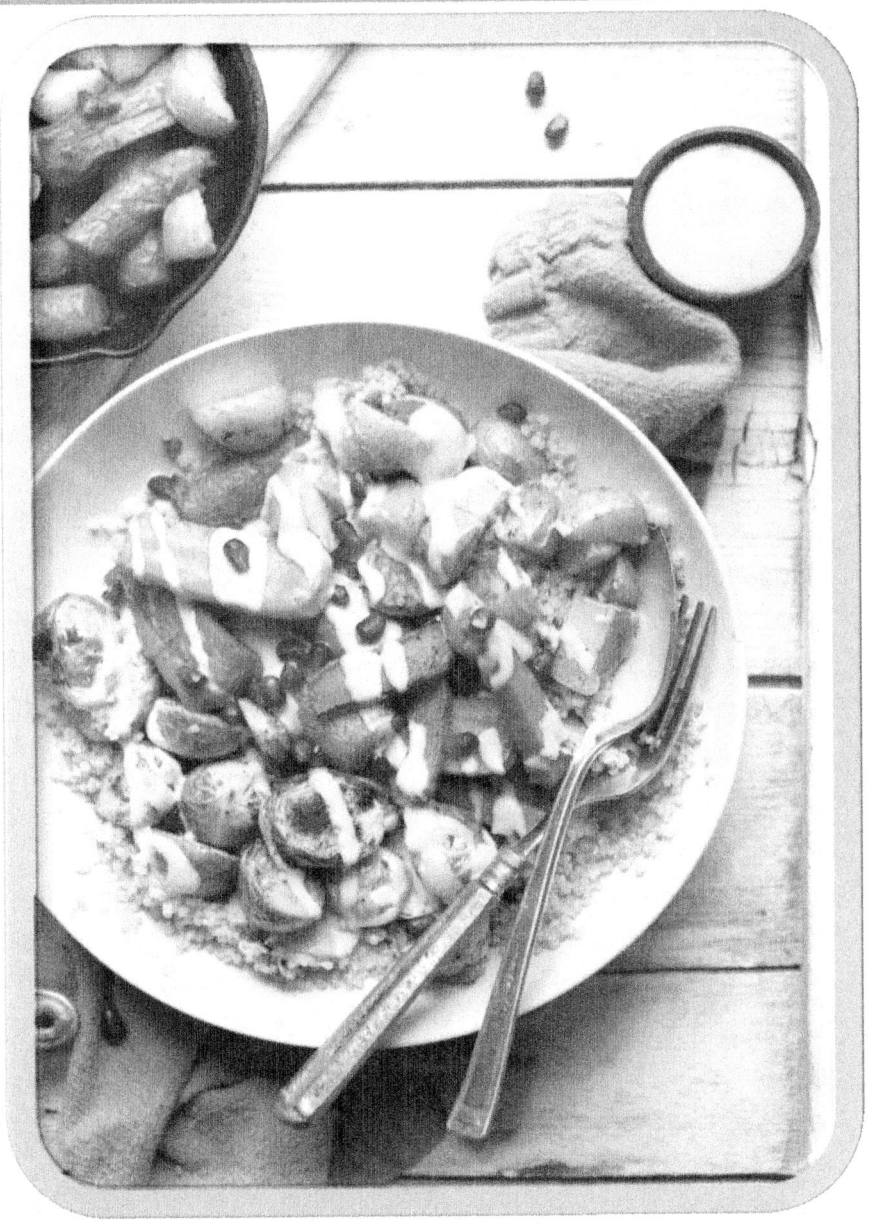

PANCAKES – 6 SMARTPOINTS®

Ingredients:

1 tsp. sweetener, artificial
1 beaten egg white
½ Tbsp. cinnamon
½ Tbsp. baking powder
½ c. buttermilk
¾ c. whole wheat flour
1/3 c. unsweetened applesauce

Directions:

1. Combine together the egg, sweetener, cinnamon, baking powder, buttermilk, flour, and applesauce inside a bowl until there are no more lumps. Add in a bit of water to help the consistency if it is too thick.
2. Spray a bit of cooking spray on the skillet and let it heat up. When the skillet is ready, add a bit of the batter to the skillet and spread it out a bit.
3. Let these pancakes cook for a few minutes to allow the bubbles to start forming.
4. At this time, flip over the pancake and let it cook for an additional minute. Take off the heat when done and then repeat the steps with the rest of the batter until done.

HEALTHY MORNING COOKIES – 2 SMARTPOINTS®

Ingredients:

2 egg whites
1/3 c. unsweetened cocoa
1/3 c. chocolate chips, mini
½ c. brown sugar, pressed down
½ c. sugar
1/8 tsp. salt
¼ c. butter, softened
1 c. flour
¼ tsp. baking soda

Directions:

1. Turn on the oven and let it heat up to 350 degrees. Take out a cookie sheet and spray it with some cooking spray.
2. Now take out a bowl and mix together the baking soda, flour, and salt. In a second bowl, combine the butter and the brown sugar and mix together until fluffy.
3. Add in the sugar to this second bowl and continue to beat to make it well incorporated. Put all of this into the flour mixture and keep on stirring to combine. Now add in the chocolate chips.
4. Place small amounts of this onto the cookie sheet and then put into the oven and let it bake for about 10 minutes.
5. Take out of the oven and allow the cookies to cool down for a few minutes before taking them off the pan and cooling down completely.

CINNAMON ROLLS—6 SMARTPOINTS

Ingredients:

¼ c. cream cheese
¼ c. sugar
¼ tsp. vanilla
1 tsp. butter, melted
11 oz. breadstick dough, cold
2 Tbsp. brown sugar
1 tsp. cinnamon

Directions:

1. Turn on the oven and let it heat up to 375 degrees. While that is heating up, take out a baking pan and prepare it with some cooking spray.
2. Take out a small bowl and mix together the brown sugar, cinnamon, and the butter and place to the side.
3. Take the breadstick dough and make it into 12 strips. Sprinkle on some brown sugar to this dough and then roll them into a spiral. Press the dough down to seal up the ends.
4. Place these rolls into a baking pan, leaving them about an inch apart. Place into the oven and let them bake for 15 minutes. When they are done, take out of the oven and let them cool for 10 minutes.
5. While the rolls are baking, work on the frosting. Bring out a bowl and mix together the cream cheese, sugar, and vanilla. Add a bit of water to this until you get the consistency that you would like.
6. Drizzle this frosting onto the prepared rolls and let it set for a few minutes before serving.

MUSHROOM AND SPINACH QUICHE – 3 SMARTPOINTS®

Ingredients:

Salt
Pepper
¼ c. chopped onion
3 eggs
½ c. cottage cheese
2 tsp. garlic, minced
1 c. artichoke hearts, chopped
½ tsp. olive oil
10 oz. spinach
1 c. mushrooms, sliced

Directions:

1. Turn on the oven and let it heat up to 350 degrees. While that is heating up, take out a pan and cook together the olive oil, mushrooms, onions, and garlic.
2. When those are ready, add in the spinach and let it cook for a bit. After a few minutes, add in the rest of the ingredients and season with some pepper and salt.
3. Place this into a prepared pie dish and let it bake for 45 minutes before serving.

APPLE MUFFIN – 7 SMARTPOINTS®

Ingredients:

½ c. milk
2 Tbsp. vegetable oil
½ tsp. salt
½ tsp. cinnamon
1 ½ tsp. baking powder
1 c. oats
½ tsp. baking soda
2/3 c. brown sugar
2 c. shredded apple
1 ½ c. flour, all purpose

Directions:

1. Turn on the oven and let it heat up to 375 degrees. In the meantime, take out a muffin pan and grease it up.
2. Take out a bowl and combine together the milk, cinnamon, vegetable oil, baking soda, salt, brown sugar, baking powder, flour, and oats.
3. When this is all combined, pour the batter inside the muffin tin and then place into the oven.
4. Allow these to bake for 18 minutes or until they are all done. Give them some time to cool down before serving.

POTATO AND CHEESE CASSEROLE – 7 SMARTPOINTS®

Ingredients:

Salt
Pepper
4 beaten eggs
1 can milk, evaporated
3 oz. bacon, chopped
½ c. scallion, sliced
3 c. potato, shredded
¾ c. cheddar cheese

Directions:

1. For this recipe, turn on the oven and let it heat up to 350 degrees. Take out your baking pan and coat it with some cooking spray.
2. Place the potatoes into the prepared baking pan and then top with some cheese, scallions, and bacon.
3. Now bring out a small bowl and mix together the pepper, salt, eggs, and milk inside. Pour this all on top of the potato mixture.
4. Place this meal inside the oven and let it cook for 40 minutes or until everything has time to set.
5. Take it out of the oven and give it a few minutes to cool down before slicing and enjoying.

CRISPY APPLE SURPRISE – 11 SMARTPOINTS®

Ingredients:
Ground cloves
- 3 lb. sliced apples
- ¼ c. sugar
- 1 tsp. vanilla
- ¼ tsp. nutmeg
- 3 Tbsp. butter
- 1 tsp. water
- ¼ tsp. cinnamon
- Salt
- ¼ c. brown sugar
- ½ tsp. ginger
- ½ c. and 2 Tbsp. flour
- ½ c. quick cooking oats

Directions;
1. For this recipe, turn on the oven and let it heat up to 375 degrees. Take out a baking dish and cover it with some cooking spray.
2. First we will need to make the topping. To do this, bring out a bowl and combine the oats with the cinnamon, salt, brown sugar, ginger, and ½ cup of flour.
3. Add in the butter at this time and then place it all into the pastry blender so that you get a nice crumbly mixture. Pour in some water and then press this to make clumps.
4. Now you will want to work on the filling. To do this, bring out a bowl and combine the cloves, sugar, nutmeg, and the rest of the flour. Put in the vanilla and the apples in as well and then pour everything inside a baking dish.
5. Pour your topping over the filling and then place everything into the oven. Bake this all in the oven for 60 minutes.

BREAKFAST JELLY PUDDING – 11 SMARTPOINTS®

Ingredients:

16 oz. fruit cocktail, canned
16 oz. mandarin orange, canned
1/3 oz. raspberry Jell-O, sugar free
20 oz. pineapple, canned
16 oz. whipped cream
1 oz. vanilla pudding mix

Directions:

1. Take out the canned fruits and take all of the liquid out of them. Bring out a bowl and combine the pudding mix, gelatin, and whipped cream.
2. Slowly fold in the fruits that you just drained out and then chill for a few hours inside the fridge before serving.

PUMPKIN MUFFINS – 4 SMARTPOINTS®

Ingredients:

18 oz. spice cake mix
15 oz. pumpkin
1 c. water

Directions:

1. For this recipe, turn on the oven and let it heat up to 375 degrees.
2. While the oven is heating up, take out a bowl and combine the water, pumpkin, and spice cake mix.
3. Prepare a muffin pan and then pour the batter inside of it. Place these into the oven and bake until it is all done before serving.

BLACKBERRY AND PEACH SMOOTHIE – 9 SMARTPOINTS®

Ingredients:

½ c. skim milk
¾ c. ice cubes
¼ c. blackberries
2 peeled peaches, sliced

Directions:

1. Bring out a blender and add in the milk, ice cubes, blackberries, and peaches.
2. Turn on the blender and let it process all of the ingredients until they are smooth.
3. Pour this into your favorite cup and then serve!

MORNING BURRITOS – 9 SMARTPOINTS®

Ingredients:

½ c. sour cream
½ c. salsa
¼ tsp. pepper
4 tortillas
2 Tbsp. cilantro
¼ tsp. salt
4 egg whites
½ c. cheddar cheese
2 chopped garlic cloves
2 eggs
1 diced green pepper
½ c. tomato, chopped
2 tsp. olive oil
1/3 c. scallions, chopped

Directions:

1. To start this recipe, turn on the oven and let it heat up to 400 degrees. Take out a baking pan and spray it with some cooking spray.
2. Now you can add in a bit of oil to the skillet and add in the tomato garlic, scallions, and green pepper. Let this cook for about 5 minutes.
3. After this time, add in the eggs and the egg whites and cook for another five minutes. Take everything off the heat at this time.
4. Add in the salt, pepper, cheese, and cilantro.
5. Lay out the tortillas and scoop a bit of the filling into each one. Roll them up tight and then place into the baking pan.
6. Bake these in the oven for 10 minutes. Serve with a bit of salsa and some sour cream and then enjoy!

BREAKFAST SOUFFLE – 3 SMARTPOINTS®

Ingredients:

1/8 tsp. cayenne pepper
2 eggs
2 egg whites
1 ½ c. cheddar cheese
½ tsp. salt
3 Tbsp. flour
1 c. milk

Directions:

1. Take out a bowl and mix three tablespoons of the milk together with the flour and set to the side.
2. Place the rest of the milk into a pan and let it cook over a low heat. Add the flour mixture to this pan and then cook it while stirring the whole time so that it can begin to thicken.
3. Remove this from the heat and then put in a bit of salt and the cayenne pepper and cheese. Move this over to a bowl and let it cool down.
4. Turn on the oven on to 350 degrees. While that is heating up, add the egg yolks into the cheese mixture until they are well incorporated.
5. Bring out a glass bowl and whip up all the egg whites together. Combine ¼ of these with the cheese mixture and then fold in the rest of the beaten egg with our rubber spatula.
6. Place this mixture into a soufflé dish and then bake in the oven for about 35 minutes. Serve right away when it is done.

BREAKFAST BARS – 6 SMARTPOINTS®

Ingredients:

1 tsp. vanilla
1/3 c. water
¾ c. chocolate chips
6 Tbsp. butter
2 egg whites
½ tsp. salt
2 c. flour
2 tsp. baking powder

Directions:

1. Turn on the oven and let it heat up to 350 degrees. While that is heating up, bring out a bowl and mix together the salt, baking powder, and flour.
2. In another bowl, mix together the butter and the brown sugar until they are nice and fluffy before adding in the egg whites and the vanilla. Slowly whisk in the flour mixture and alternate it with a bit of water as well.
3. Add in the chocolate chips and mix them in well. Place some foil onto a baking pan and then pour the mixture on the pan.
4. Place this into the oven and let it bake for 25 minutes. Let the bars cool on a wire rack when you are done. Cut into slices when you are ready and enjoy.

FRENCH TOAST – 3 SMARTPOINTS®

Ingredients:

6 slices wheat bread
1 pkg. sugar free maple syrup
1 Tbsp. cinnamon
1 Tbsp. vanilla
Cooking spray
4 egg whites
¼ c. skim milk

Directions:

1. To start this recipe, bring out a bowl and mix together the egg whites and the vanilla.
2. Take out a skillet and grease it u with some cooking spray. Heat up the skillet.
3. While the skillet is heating up, dip the bread slices in the egg mixture and let each side get nice and soaked. Allow the extra batter to drip off.
4. Place the bread onto the skillet and let each side cook for about 3 minutes. Place these onto a plate and serve.

CHEESE AND HAM OMELET – 6 SMARTPOINTS®

Ingredients:

½ c. diced ham
¼ c. Parmesan cheese
1/8 tsp. pepper
1/8 tsp. hot pepper sauce
2 Tbsp. green onion, chopped
¼ tsp. salt
2 eggs
4 egg whites

Directions:

1. For this recipe, bring out a bowl and ix together the hot sauce, salt, pepper, eggs, and onion.
2. Take out a skillet and grease it with some cooking spray before heating it up. Pour the mixture into the skillet and let it cook for 5 minutes so it has time to set.
3. Sprinkle the top with the ham and the Parmesan cheese. Fold the omelet in half and let it cook for another minute before serving.

SPICED HONEY CAKE – 7 SMARTPOINTS®

Ingredients:

- 1 tsp. grated orange zest
- 2 Tbsp. canola oil
- ½ c. honey
- ¼ c. sliced almonds
- 2 eggs
- ¼ c. white sugar
- ½ tsp. nutmeg
- ½ tsp. cloves
- 1 tsp. cinnamon
- ¾ tsp. allspice
- ½ tsp. baking soda
- 1/8 tsp. salt
- 1 ½ c. flour
- ¾ tsp. baking powder
- ½ c. applesauce

Directions:

1. To start this recipe, turn on the oven and let it heat up to 350 degrees. Grease up a loaf pan using some cooking spray and set it to the side.
2. Mix together the nutmeg, cloves, cinnamon, allspice, baking soda, salt, four, and baking powder. When this is combined, set it aside.
3. In another bowl, beat together the eggs until they are frothy. Add in the sugar, honey, and oil and mix to make this a pale yellow before adding in the orange zest and apple sauce.
4. Slowly combined in the wet mixture and the dry mixture, making sure to combine them together well. When these are read, pour inside a loaf pan and then top with some almonds.
5. Place all of this into the oven and let it bake for about 40 minutes until it is cooked all the way through.
6. Allow the cake to cool down for another 20 minutes before serving.

BLUEBERRY MUFFINS – 5 SMARTPOINTS®

Ingredients:

2 ½ c. hot water
1 ½ tsp. baking powder
3 c. bran cereal
19 oz. blueberry muffin mix

Directions:

1. Turn on the oven and let it heat up to 400 degrees. Prepare a muffin pan using some paper liners or with some cooking spray.
2. While the oven is heating up, combine the hot water and the bran cereal together and then set them to the side.
3. Bring out another bowl so that you can mix together the baking powder and the muffin mix. When these are combined, place the bran cereal and water so that they can be incorporated as well.
4. Pour this batter inside of your prepared muffin pan and then bake for 15 minutes or until the muffins are cooked all the way through.

YOGURT FLUFF – 2 SMARTPOINTS®

Ingredients:

12 tsp. vanilla
Ice cubes
½ c. cold water
1 c. yogurt
¾ c. boiling water
8 ½ grams cherry gelatin

Directions:

1. Combine together the gelatin and the boiling water inside of a bowl and ix so that the gelatin is completely dissolved.
2. Put the ice cubes into some cold water and then get a cup of this mixture. Pour this into the gelatin and continue to mix so that it can become thicker. Get rid of any ice that is extra.
3. Add in the yogurt as well as the vanilla and let it stir until it becomes well blended.
4. Place the bowl into the fridge and let it chill for at least 30 minutes. After this time add in some whipped cream and enjoy!

WEIGHT WATCHERS LUNCHES

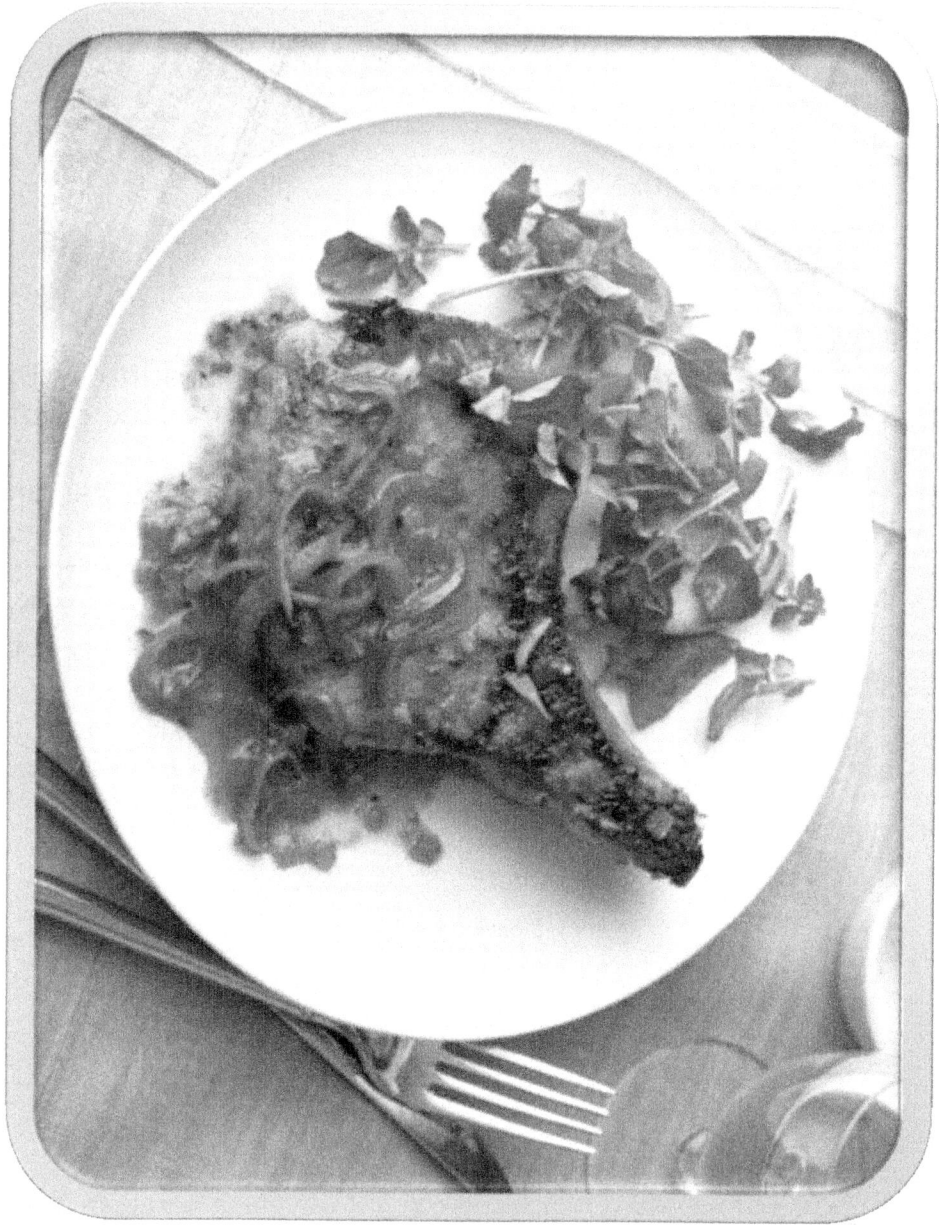

CREAMY PESTO PASTA – 7 SMARTPOINTS®

Ingredients:

1 tsp. lemon juice
1 ½ tsp. olive oil
2 ½ Tbsp. cream cheese
2 garlic cloves
4 ½ c. baby spinach
2 Tbsp. water
1 ¼ tsp. salt
8 oz. uncooked spaghetti

Directions:

1. For this recipe, take out a pot of water and boil it with a bit of salt. Add in the pasta and let it cook for 8 minutes or until it is all done.
2. Drain out the water and top with some cherry tomatoes and Parmesan cheese. Process the salt, oil, garlic, spinach, and water inside the blender until it is soft.
3. Add in the cream cheese to the pasta until it melts. Then add in the reserved pasta water and the pesto sauce and mix to get the right consistency.
4. Season with some lemon juice and salt and then enjoy.

BBQ PORK SANDWICH – 5 SMARTPOINTS®

Ingredients:
1 cut bell pepper, green
6 hamburger buns
12 oz. pork tenderloin
¼ tsp. salt
1 tsp. Worcestershire sauce
1 Tbsp. brown sugar

1 ½ tsp. chili powder
6 oz. can tomato paste
2 Tbsp. red wine vinegar
2 minced garlic cloves
2/3 c. water
1 minced onion

Directions:

1. Grease up a small pan with some cooking spray and then heat it up. Add in the onion and the garlic and let these cook for 5 minutes.
2. At this time, add in the oregano, Worcestershire sauce, brown sugar, chili powder, tomato paste, vinegar, and garlic. Bring all of this to a boil.
3. Simmer this without the top on for about 10 minutes so that the liquid can reduce a bit, making sure to stir occasionally.
4. While that is cooking, take the meat and remove the fat a bit. Cut this meat into smaller strips. Take out another skillet and brush with some cooking spray.
5. Season the meat with some salt and place the meat in the skillet. Cook the meat for three minutes before pouring in the bell peppers and sauce.
6. Cook all of the ingredients together for a few minutes. When it is ready, serve the pork on toasted buns and enjoy.

ITALIAN CHICKEN – 5 SMARTPOINTS®

Ingredients:

Juice from two lemons
Pepper
Salt
2 Tbsp. capers
¼ c. parsley, chopped
½ c. chicken broth
2 Tbsp. butter
1 ½ lbs. chicken breast, sliced
¾ c. white wine

Directions:

1. To start up this recipe, turn on the oven and let it heat up to 350 degrees. Lay out the chicken breasts onto a board and then cover with some cling wrap. Flatten the chicken with a mallet to make them ¼ inch thick.
2. Season the chicken with the pepper and salt and then move this over to a baking dish. Add some butter to the chicken and then surround it with the broth, wine, and lemon juice.
3. Sprinkle everything with the capers and then cover with some foil before placing into the oven and baking for 20 minutes.
4. Remove the foil after this time and then bake them for an additional 10 minutes. Sprinkle with some parsley and then serve right away.

BAKED TORTELLINI – 6 SMARTPOINTS®

Ingredients:

2/3 c. mozzarella cheese	2 Tbsp. flour
2 tsp. lemon zest	2 c. milk
2 c. spinach	2 bacon slices
¼ tsp. red pepper flakes	3 chopped garlic cloves
1 Tbsp. lemon juice	12 oz. dry spinach and cheese
1/8 tsp. pepper	
1 ½ tsp. basil	1 pkg. tortellini
¾ tsp. salt	1 ½ oz. Parmesan cheese

Directions:

1. Turn on the oven and let it heat up to 350 degrees. While that is heating up, take out a baking dish and cover with some cooking spray.
2. Follow the directions on the package and cook the tortellini. In the meantime, place the bacon into a skillet and cook for 9 minutes so it becomes crisp. Take the bacon off the skillet and put on a paper towel to absorb the oil. Save some of this bacon grease.
3. Add the garlic into the bacon grease and let it cook for a minute before adding in the flour and whisk in the milk. Now add in the basil, red pepper flakes, and pepper.
4. Bring all of this to a simmer and then add in the lemon juice and lemon zest and let t stir for another 3 minutes.
5. Take all of this off the heat. Crumble up the bacon and set it to the side. Mix the mozzarella, spinach, parmesan, and tortellini together.
6. Move this mixture to the baking dish and top with the rest of the bacon, Parmesan, and mozzarella.
7. Cover this with foil and place into the oven to bake for 20 minutes. Remove the foil at this time and then bake for another 10 minutes before serving.

CHEESY MUSHROOMS – 2 SMARTPOINTS®

Ingredients:

½ tsp. olive oil
1/8 tsp. cayenne pepper
1 tsp. lemon juice
½ tsp. lemon zest
2 Tbsp. feta cheese
½ Tbsp. parsley
8 mushrooms
2 pieces mushroom stems

Directions:

1. Turn on the oven and let it heat up to 425 degrees. Bring out a baking dish and let it get covered with cooking spray.
2. Rinse the mushrooms and dry them with some paper towels. Pull the stems off the mushrooms and set two of these to the side. Mince up the mushroom stems and place into a bowl.
3. Place the mushrooms into the baking dish and then mx in the rest of the ingredients with the minced stems. Place this mixture into the caps of the mushrooms.
4. Place this into the oven and let it bake for about 15 minutes. Allow this some time to cool down before serving.

BAKED BURRITO – 6 SMARTPOINTS®

Ingredients:

¼ c. water
1 c. Mexican cheese
10 oz. canned refried beans
1 c. Bisquick
1 c. mozzarella cheese
1 lb. ground beef
1 pack taco seasoning

Directions:

1. Cook up the ground beef and until it is cooked all the way through and then drain out the liquid. Add in the taco seasoning and let it simmer.
2. Bring out another bowl and combine the refried beans with the Bisquick and water. Put this mixture into a pan and then top with some cheese and beef.
3. Turn on the oven to 350 degrees and then add in the meal. Bake this for 30 minutes and then serve.

ITALIAN BREAD WITH SOME TUNA SALAD – 10 SMARTPOINTS®

Ingredients:

8 oz. Italian bread
2 tomatoes, sliced
¼ tsp. salt
1 tsp. dried oregano
½ tsp. pepper
3 Tbsp. balsamic vinegar
1 red onion, sliced
1 Tbsp. capers, rinsed or drained.
4 c. lettuce, shredded
8 oz. white tuna

Directions:

1. Start by making the tuna salad part. Mix together the onion, capers, lettuce, and tuna. Set this to the side.
2. Then you can go on and make the dressing. To do this, you will be able to mix together the salt, pepper, garlic, oregano, vinegar, olive oil. Drizzle this on top of the tuna salad and toss around to combine.
3. Next it is time to make the sandwiches. You can cut the bread lengthwise and then spread it open. Arrange the tomatoes on the bottom of the bread.
4. Top this all with the salad mixture and then wrap up the sandwich with some cling wrap. Chill in the fridge for a few hours before serving.

TURKEY AND CHEESE SANDWICH – 10 SMARTPOINTS®

Ingredients:

8 slices of bread
4 oz. sliced cheese
½ c. milk
4 tsp. Dijon mustard
4 oz. sliced chicken breast
1 egg
1 egg white

Directions:

1. Take out a small bowl and whisk together the milk, egg, and egg white. Lay out the bread and layer with some of the mustard on top.
2. Top the bread slices with some turkey and cheese. Put the rest of the bread slices on top of them to put the sandwiches together.
3. Grease a pan with some cooking spray and then place over the heat. Coat each of the sandwiches with the egg mixture and place inside a hot pan.
4. Cook the sandwiches for about 4 minutes on each side before serving.

VEGGIE SOUP – 1 SMARTPOINT

Ingredients:

1 tsp. Cajun spices
¼ tsp. basil
2 beef bouillon cubs
½ c. zucchini slices
2 minced garlic cloves
14 ½ oz. canned tomatoes, diced
2 ½ c. cabbage, shredded
1 ½ stalks chopped celery
14 oz. canned beef broth
½ sliced onion
1 c. sliced carrot

Directions:

1. Spray a pan with some cooking spray and then add inn the celery, onions, and carrots inside.
2. Take out a big pot and mx together the basil, garlic, Cajun spice, cabbage, bouillon cubes, beef broth, and tomatoes together. Add in the vegetables you just cooked as well.
3. Bring all of this to a boil and let it simmer together for about 30 minutes.
4. After this time, put the zucchini into the pot and simmer for an additional 10 minutes. Serve it warm.

CHEESEBURGER SOUP – 7 SMARTPOINTS®

Ingredients:
1/8 tsp. pepper
24 pieces corn tortilla chips
½ tsp. paprika
¼ tsp. salt
1 c. evaporated milk
8 oz. cubed Velveeta
Cooking spray

2 Tbsp. flour
3 c. chicken broth
1 chopped celery stalk
1 lb. uncooked ground beef
1 chopped garlic clove
1 diced onion

Directions:
1. Take out a skillet and spray on some cooking spray. Add on the celery, garlic, and onion and let these cook until they are tender.
2. Bring out a slow cooker and spray with some cooking spray. Transfer these over to the slow cooker.
3. Take out another skillet and cook the beef for about six minutes or until it is cooked through. Move this over to the slow cooker.
4. In another bowl, mix together ½ cup of the broth so that you can get rid of the lumps. Put the flour into the skillet and add in the rest 2 ½ cups of broth inside.
5. Let this simmer, taking time to take the browned bits off the bottom of the skillet. When this is done, move it over to the slow cooker and add in the pepper, paprika, salt, evaporated milk, and cheese.
6. Place the lid into the slow cooker and let it cook on a low setting for 2 hours. Pour your flour mixture inside the slow cooker at this time.
7. Cover the slow cooker and let this cook for another 15 minutes. When you are ready to serve, add some crushed tortilla chips and enjoy.

PASTA VEGGIES – 5 SMARTPOINTS®

Ingredients:

½ c. mayo
2 Tbsp. scallions, sliced
½ tsp. red pepper
¼ c. celery, diced
¾ c. salsa
½ yellow bell pepper
½ c. cherry tomatoes
6 oz. pasta
12 oz. tuna, canned

Directions:

1. Cook the pasta by following the directions on the package. When this is done, drain out the pasta and rinse it under some cold water. Then drain it again.
2. Now you can bring out a big bowl and mix together the celery, bell pepper, tomatoes, pasta, and tuna.
3. In a second bowl, combine the red pepper, salsa, and mayo together. Pour this dressing over the pasta mixture and toss it together well.
4. Cover the bowl and then place into the fridge to chill for a bit. Right before serving, top with some scallions and enjoy.

BACON WRAP – 8 SMARTPOINTS®

Ingredients:

½ lb. sliced roast beef
2 sliced tomatoes
¼ tsp. pepper
7 pieces tortilla
2 tsp. Dijon mustard
2 c. shredded lettuce
¼ tsp. salt
1/3 c. basil
1/3 c. mayo

Directions:

1. Bring out a bowl and combine the pepper, Dijon mustard, salt, basil, and mayo.
2. Lay out the tortillas and spread the mixture from above all over it.
3. Sprinkle the tortillas with some lettuce, roast beef, and tomatoes. Roll this up and then serve.

BAKED FISH – 5 SMARTPOINTS®

Ingredients:

½ tsp. paprika
1/3 c. milk
½ tsp. salt
3 Tbsp. melted butter
1/8 tsp. pepper
¼ c. bread crumbs
½ tsp. dill
1 ½ lb. white fish fillet
¼ c. yellow cornmeal

Directions:

1. Turn on the oven and let it heat up to 450 degrees. Bring out a pie plate and combine together all of your dry ingredients.
2. Add in the milk to another milk. Dip the fish inside the milk to coat and then put it through the crumb mixture.
3. Place the fish into a greased pan and then drizzle the fish with some melted butter.
4. Bake the fish for 10 minutes and then serve with your favorite sides.

BEEF ZITI BAKE – 7 SMARTPOINTS®

Ingredients:
20 oz. crushed tomatoes
1 c. mozzarella cheese
1 tsp. oregano
1 tsp. thyme
¼ tsp. pepper
1/3 lb. ground beef
½ tsp. salt
2 minced garlic cloves
12 oz. ziti
2 tsp. olive oil
Directions:
1. Turn on the oven and let it heat up to 350 degrees. Cook the ziti by following the directions on the package. When this is done, drain out the pasta and rinse it off.
2. Heat up some olive oil into a pan and then cook the garlic inside for a minute. Cook the ground beef in here, seasoning with some pepper and salt, and cook all the way through.
3. Remove the fat and then mix in the thyme, rosemary, and oregano and cook for two more minutes. Add in the tomatoes and bring to a boil to simmer for five minutes.
4. Bring out a casserole dish and put some of the meat sauce to cover all of the bottom. Put in half of your prepared ziti and then the rest of the meat sauce. Now add in half of the mozzarella cheese and then finish the layers.
5. Bake the ziti in the oven for 30 minutes so the cheese has time to melt the cheese before serving.

CHICKEN SALAD – 4 SMARTPOINTS®

Ingredients:

½ tsp. salt
¼ tsp. pepper
1 tsp. Dijon mustard
1 tsp. lemon juice
2 Tbsp. sour cream
2 Tbsp. parsley
1/3 c. dill pickle
¼ c. mayo
1 lb. chicken breast
½ c. celery, chopped

Directions:

1. Take out a pan and place the chicken inside. Add in just enough water to cover up the chicken. Bring this all to a boil.
2. Allow the chicken to boil for 10 minutes and then drain out the liquid, allowing the chicken to cool a bit.
3. Slice the chicken into small cubes and then place the chicken into a bowl.
4. At this time, add in the pepper, salt, lemon juice, parsley, mustard, mayo, sour cream, celery, and pickles together. Toss around to coat and serve.

EGG SALAD – 4 SMARTPOINTS®

Ingredients:

¼ tsp. pepper
½ tsp. salt
1 piece of dill
2 Tbsp. mayo
½ tsp. Dijon mustard
2 Tbsp. chives
4 eggs
2 hard boiled eggs

Directions:

1. Bring out a pan and fill it with the water and the eggs. Place this on a high heat and bring it to a boil.
2. When the eggs are done, drain the water out and add in the eggs to an ice water bath. When the eggs are cooled down, you can remove the shells from the eggs.
3. Also take some time to remove the yolks from two the eggs. Slice up the eggs into smaller pieces and add into a bowl.
4. Add in the pepper, salt, mustard, dill, chives, and mayo to the bowl and stir well before serving.

BEEF BURGERS – 4 SMARTPOINTS®

Ingredients;

½ tsp. salt
¼ tsp. pepper
Four hamburger buns, low calorie
1 Tbsp. Worcestershire sauce
2 tsp. garlic, minced
Cooking spray
1 lb. ground beef

Directions:

1. Coat your griddle with some cooking spray and heat it up. Take out a bowl and add in the pepper, salt, Worcestershire sauce, garlic, and beef. Form this into patties.
2. Place the burgers onto the prepared griddle and cook the patties for five minutes on each side.
3. Add some of our favorite toppings and then enjoy.

WEIGHT WATCHERS DINNERS RECIPES

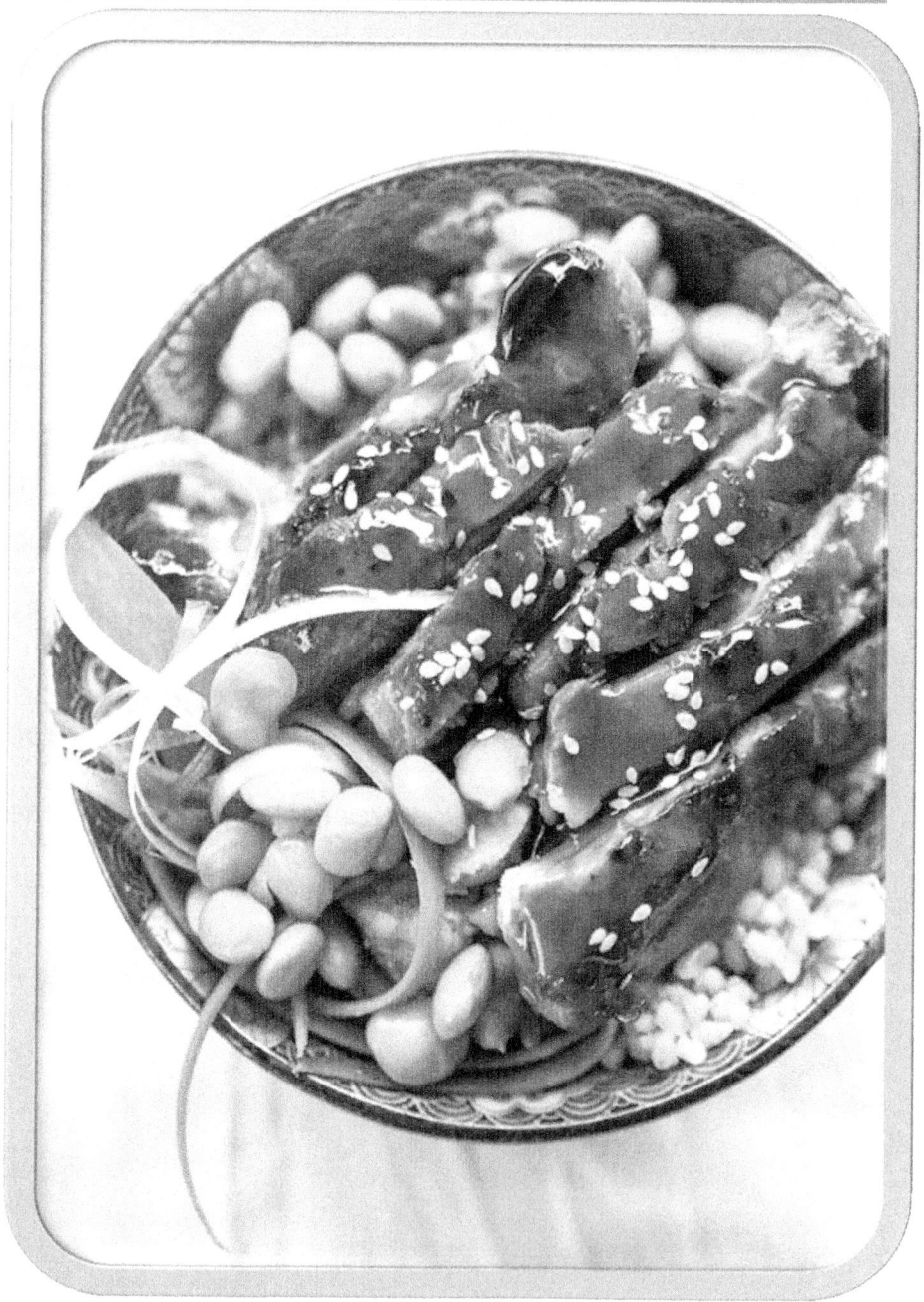

CHEESY CHICKEN CHOPS == 3 SMART POINTS

Ingredients:

½ tsp. garlic powder
¼ tsp. pepper
1 lb. chicken breast
1/8 tsp. paprika
1 tsp. parsley
¼ c. parmesan cheese
2 Tbsp. dried Italian bread crumbs

Directions:

1. Turn on the oven and let it heat up to 400 degrees. Bring out a bag and add in the seasonings, cheese, and crumbs and mix them together.
2. Move this mixture over to a plate. Coat the chicken in this cheese mixture and then move over to a baking sheet.
3. Allow this to bake inside the air fryer for about 25 minutes or until it is cooked through and then serve.

JALAPENO CHICKEN – 5 SMARTPOINTS®

Ingredients:

2 Tbsp. Worcestershire sauce
16 oz. chicken breasts
1 tsp. garlic powder
1/3 c. steak sauce
1/3 c. jalapeno jelly, melted

Directions:

1. Bring out a small bowl and mix together the Worcestershire sauce, garlic powder, steak sauce, and jalapeno jelly.
2. Add the chicken into this mixture and let it marinate inside the fridge overnight.
3. Spray the griddle with some cooking spray. Cook the chicken for about 5 minutes on each side so that the chicken can cook through.

CILANTRO LIME SHRIMP – 3 SMARTPOINTS®

Ingredients:

¼ tsp. pepper
¼ c. cilantro, chopped
1 tsp. lime zest, grated
2 minced garlic cloves
1 Tbsp. olive oil
½ tsp. cumin
¼ tsp. ginger
1 ¾ lb. shrimp
2 Tbsp. lime juice
½ tsp. salt

Directions;

1.　To make this simple recipe, bring out a bowl and mix together the garlic, cumin, ginger, shrimp, and lime juice.
2.　Heat up some oil inside a skillet and then add in the shrimp. Let it cook inside the skillet for about 4 minutes.
3.　Before serving, garnish with some pepper, salt, cilantro, and lime zest.

SPINACH AND CHICKEN CRESCENTS == 4 SMARTPOINTS®

Ingredients:

1 c. baby spinach
1/3 c. Mexican blend cheese
5 oz. chicken strips, grilled
8 oz. crescent roll dough
4 Tbsp. cream cheese, soft

Directions:

1. Turn on the oven and let it heat up to 375 degrees. Put the crescent rolls onto a baking sheet and put some spinach and cream cheese on top of the rolls.
2. Grill up the chicken strips if you need to and then place these on the crescent with the Mexican cheese.
3. Tuck in the roll to wrap up the filling and then bake the meal for about 14 minutes inside the oven before serving.

STEAK AND MASHED POTATOES – 8 SMARTPOINTS®

Ingredients;

1 ½ c. beef broth
4 cube steaks
Pepper
8 oz. sliced mushrooms
4 Tbsp. flour
1 lb. diced potatoes
½ tsp. salt

Directions:

1. To start this recipe, bring out a pot and boil and simmer the potatoes until they are nice and tender. Drain these out when you are done and keep ½ cup of the liquid.
2. Season the cooked potatoes with some pepper and salt and then mash them up using the liquid that you reserved.
3. Mix together some of the extra liquid with 2 tablespoon flour. Cover the steaks with the remaining flour as well as some salt and pepper and then cook the steaks for about 2 minutes on each side.
4. Mix in the mushrooms to this mixture and bring it all to a boil. When it reaches a boil, simmer the ingredients for 30 minutes.
5. Remove the cover at this time and cook so the gravy can thicken. Serve with some of the mashed potatoes and enjoy.

HONEY SALMON – 4 SMARTPOINTS®

Ingredients:

½ tsp. pepper
¼ c. sliced scallions
1 lb. salmon fillets
½ tsp. salt
1 tsp. ginger
2 tsp. wasabi
1 Tbsp. soy sauce
1 Tbsp. honey
3 Tbsp. mirin
1 Tbsp. rice vinegar

Direction:

1. Boil the wasabi, ginger, soy sauce, honey, mirin, and vinegar together in a pan for about five minutes.
2. After this time, take it off the heat and sprinkle with some salt and pepper. Sprinkle with a bit of salt and pepper.
3. Grease up a skillet and let it heat up a little bit. Cook the salmon in the skillet on 4 minutes on both sides.
4. Spoon a bit of the sauce on top of the salmon and then top a bit of the scallions on top of it before serving.

VEGGIE PORK CHOPS – 6 SMARTPOINTS®

Ingredients:

1 ½ tsp. oregano
½ tsp. cumin
2 c. corn
½ c. salsa
1 diced onion
14.5 oz. can stewed tomatoes
16 oz. pork chops
1 diced green peppers

Directions:

1. Turn the oven on and let it heat up to 350 degrees. Cook up the pork chops in a preheated skillet and let it cook for two minutes on each side of the meat.
2. Move the pork over to a prepared casserole dish. Grease up the skillet with some more cooking spray and then add in the rest of the ingredients. Cook these for about five minutes.
3. When these ingredients are well combined, pour this mixture all over the pork chops and then cover the dish with some foil.
4. Bake the pork chops in the oven for about 50 minutes or until the pork is cooked through before serving.

MEXICAN CASSEROLE – 8 SMARTPOINTS®

Ingredients:

1/3 c. Mexican cheese blend
1/3 chopped cilantro bunch
8 pieces corn tortilla
¾ c. sour cream
15 oz. corn kernels
15 oz. can black beans
¼ c. jalapeno pepper, chopped
2 c. tomato, chopped
1 lb. ground beef
½ c. diced onion

Directions:

1. Bring out our skillet and cook the onions and beef inside for about 12 minutes. Drain and rinse off the meat with some warm water in order to remove some of the fat.
2. Place the meat into the skillet again and add in the taco seasoning mix, tomatoes, jalapenos, corn, and black beans and let this heat and simmer for another five minutes.
3. Cut the 8 tortillas in half and then arrange 8 of the halves into a prepared baking dish. Put half of the beef mixture and the sour cream over the tortillas.
4. Cover with the rest of the tortillas and then the rest of the beef mixture. Turn the oven on to 350 degrees at this time.
5. Bake the dish for about 25 minutes. When this is all done, top with some cilantro and cheese before serving.

CHICKEN THAI WRAP – 2 SMARTPOINTS®

Ingredients:

½ tsp. grated ginger
1 handful sliced green onions
½ tsp. soy sauce
Hot sauce
1/3 c. cabbage
¼ c. snap peas
1/3 c. red bell pepper strips
2 Tbsp. PB2
1 wheat wrap
2 oz. chicken breast

Directions:

1. Start this recipe by bringing out a bowl and mixing together the green onions and the PB2.
2. Then take out a plate and heat up the tortillas inside of the microwave for about 20 seconds.
3. Place the dressing on top of the tortilla and then add in the vegetables and chicken. Wrap up the tortilla and then enjoy.

PITA BREAD PIZZA – 9 SMARTPOINTS®

Ingredients:

2 tsp. Parmesan cheese
Pinch of pizza seasoning
10 chopped black olives
½ c. mozzarella cheese
¼ c. mushrooms, sliced
¼ c. green pepper
1 pita bread
¼ c. pizza sauce

Directions:

1. Lay out the pita bread and put the pizza sauce all over it. Top this with the seasoning, mozzarella, parmesan cheese, and vegetables.
2. Spray this with a bit of cooking spray and then place it on a baking pan. Turn on the oven to broil.
3. Put the pita into the oven and let it broil in the oven for 2 minutes to let the cheese melt. Take it out of the oven and let it cool down for a bit before serving.

POTATO SOUP – 4 SMARTPOINTS®

Ingredients:

1 c. water
6 Tbsp. bacon bits
1 pack of gravy
1 c. skim milk
32 oz. hash browns, non-fat
3 cans chicken broth

Directions:

1. Bring out a pot and coat it with some cooking spray. Heat it up and then add in the hash browns.
2. After a few minutes, add in the chicken broth and bring this to a boil before lowering the heat and letting this come to a simmer.
3. While the hash browns are heating up, take out another bowl and mix together the gravy mix, water, and milk.
4. Pour this mixture in with the cooked potatoes and then add in the bacon bits. Cook this for a little bit longer to allow it time to thicken. Season with some salt and then serve.

ROAST BEEF WITH VEGGIES – 8 SMARTPOINTS®

Ingredients:

14 oz. diced tomatoes
1 pack onion soup mix
4 carrots, chunked
1 onion, quartered
2 roast beef
2 lbs. wedged potatoes

Directions:

1. Place the roast into your slow cooker and then top it with the onion soup mix.
2. When that is organized, add in the carrots, onion, and potatoes and then top with the tomatoes.
3. Place the cover onto the slow cooker and let this cook on a low setting for about 7 hours.

MUSHROOM STEAK – 5 SMARTPOINTS®

Ingredients:
2 tsp. Worcestershire sauce
Parsley
2 Tbsp. flour
2 Tbsp. tomato paste
1/8 tsp. pepper
8 oz. sliced mushrooms
2 c. beef broth
¼ tsp. salt
1 egg
1 egg white
1 lb. ground turkey
½ c. bread crumbs
1 ½ tsp. cooking oil
¾ c. onions, minced
½ tsp. mustard powder
¼ c. water
1 tsp. red wine vinegar

Directions:

1. Take out a skillet and cook the oil and the onions together for about 5 minutes.
2. Bring out a bowl and mix together the black pepper, salt, egg, egg white, ground turkey, bread crumbs, half of the cooked onions, ¼ cup of the beef broth, and the ground beef.
3. When this is all combined, use our hands to form these into 8 patties. Add into the skillet and cook on each side to brown.
4. Add the pepper, salt, and mushrooms into the skillet and cook for another 3 minutes. Then add the patties back inside.
5. While that is cooking, mix together the broth and the flour. Then add in the Worcestershire sauce, mustard powder, vinegar, water, tomato paste, and the rest of the onions.
6. Pour this sauce over the meat and mushrooms in the skillet. Serve it warm.

CHEESE AND TUNA SANDWICH – 10 SMARTPOINTS®

Ingredients:

1 sliced tomato
½ c. cheddar cheese
1 ½ Tbsp. butter
2 Tbsp. spicy brown mustard
1 ½ Tbsp. pickle relish
4 slices bread
5 oz. can tuna
1 ½ Tbsp. mayo

Directions:

1. Bring out a bowl and combine together the pickle relish, drained tuna, and the mayo.
2. Lay out the bread and spread out some butter on one of the slices and then mustard on the other.
3. Put the cheese, tomato, and tuna on the side with the mustard and then place the other two slices on top to make our sandwich.
4. Place these both into a pan and then cover and cook for 3 minutes on both sides. Cut in half and then enjoy!

COLA CHICKEN – 5 SMARTPOINTS®

Ingredients:

1 can of diet cola
½ c. onion, chopped
4 chicken breasts, skinless
1 c. ketchup

Directions:

1. Bring out a skillet to start this recipe and combine the cola and the ketchup inside.
2. After a few minutes, add in the chicken and the onions and stir it all around. Bring this to a boil before placing the cover on top and reducing the heat.
3. Simmer the whole meal together for about 45 minutes so that the chicken has time to marinate before serving.

BEEF CHILI – 4 SMARTPOINTS®

Ingredients:

2 Tbsp. tomato paste
Pepper
1 chopped sweet onion
¼ c. diced green chilies
28 oz. tomatoes in a can
15 oz. red kidney beans,
2 Tbsp. chili powder
2 tsp. cumin
1 diced red bell pepper
1 diced green bell pepper
1 lb. ground turkey or beef
1 Tbsp. minced garlic

Directions:

1. To start this recipe, bring out a skillet and brown the ground beef together with the garlic. When these are done cooking, take the fat out of the skillet and then add in the bell peppers.
2. Cook this for 5 minutes so that the peppers can get nice and soft. Now add in the chili powder and cumin and cook for a few more minutes.
3. Bring out a slow cooker and add in the meat mixture, tomato paste, chilies, onion, tomatoes, and kidney beans inside.
4. Put the lid on top of the slow cooker and let this cook for about 5 hours. When you are ready to serve, season with some black pepper and serve.

VEGETABLE QUESADILLA – 9 SMARTPOINTS®

Ingredients:

Cooking spray
¼ c. shredded cheddar cheese
¼ c. shredded mozzarella cheese
Salt
2 wheat flour tortillas
1 dash cayenne pepper
Pepper
1 Tbsp. red bell pepper, diced
1 tsp. soy sauce
1/3 c. shredded carrot
1/3 c. broccoli, chopped
½ Tbsp. canola oil
½ c. mushrooms, sliced

Directions:

1. To start this recipe, bring out a pan and cook up the vegetables inside for 7 minutes to make it nice and soft. Season with the salt, soy sauce, and the peppers.
2. When the vegetables are all done cooking place them into the bowl.
3. Clean out the pan if needed and place one of the tortillas inside. Top with half the cheese, some vegetables, and then the remainder of the cheese. Place the second tortilla on top.
4. Heat this for about 2 minutes to make it nice and warm. After that time, turn the quesadilla over and let it cook for another minute before serving.

BAKED CHICKEN – 10 SMARTPOINTS®

Ingredients:
2 Tbsp. Worcestershire sauce
2 tsp. dry mustard
3 Tbsp. brown sugar
2 Tbsp. vinegar
4 chicken breasts
½ c. ketchup

Directions:
1. Turn on the oven and let it heat up to 350 degrees.
2. While the oven is heating up, place the chicken into the baking dish and then add in the ketchup, vinegar, brown sugar, dry mustard, and Worcestershire sauce all around the chicken.
3. Place these into the oven and bake the meal for 40 minutes. Allow some time to cool down before serving.

CHICKEN AND DUMPLINGS – 9 SMARTPOINTS®

Ingredients:
Tortillas
Pepper
Salt
½ Tbsp. celery salt
3 c. chicken breast, chopped
2 cans chicken broth
1 can cream of chicken soup

Directions:
1. Take out a pan and add together the chicken breast, cream of chicken soup, and chicken broth. Sprinkle in the seasonings.
2. Add the tortillas one at a time. Reduce the heat and let it simmer for 25 minutes.

SMART POINTS SLOW COOKER RECIPES

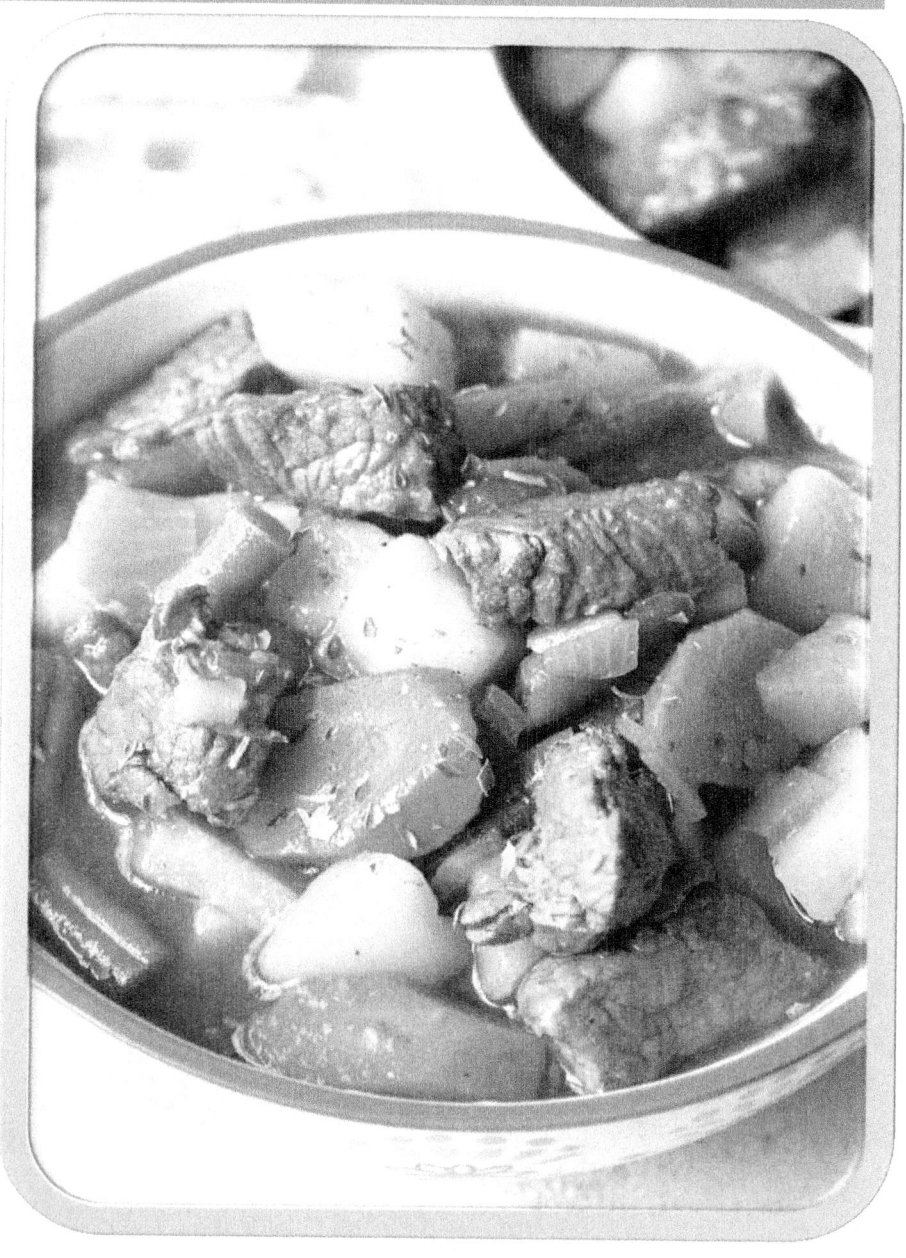

SLOW COOKED BEEF AND BARBEQUE

This recipe needs 10 minutes to prepare, 6 hours to cook and will make 8 servings.

Each serving contains
- Protein: 25 grams
- Carbs: 17 grams
- Fats: 16.8 grams
- Saturated Fats: 1.2 grams
- Sugar: 8.7 grams
- Fiber .5 grams
- Calories: 313
- Smart Points: 9

What to Use
- Ground black pepper (to taste)
- Sea salt (to taste)
- Cayenne pepper (.25 tsp.)
- Paprika (1 tsp.)
- Garlic powder (1 tsp.)
- Onion powder (1 T)
- Worcestershire sauce (2 tsp.)
- Hot sauce (1 T)
- Brown sugar (.5 cups)
- Yellow mustard (.5 cups)
- Ketchup (1 cup)
- Apple cider vinegar (1 cup)
- Beef roast (2 lbs.)

What to Do

1. Add 1 cup of water as well as the beef to a slow cooker and let them cook, covered, on a low setting for 6 hours.
2. Once the ingredients are done cooking, discard the bones and add everything else to a blender and blend well prior to serving.
3. At the 5 hour mark, start to prepare the barbeque sauce by taking a saucepan and adding gin the cayenne, paprika, garlic powder, onion powder, Worcestershire sauce, hot sauce, brown sugar, yellow mustard, ketchup and apple cider vinegar and mixing well before placing it on top of a burner over a stove set to a high heat.
4. Let the sauce boil 5 minutes, regularly stirring.
5. After the slow cooker, has finished cooking the beef, remove it and drain the slow cooker before adding in the beef as well as 60 percent of the sauce.
6. Cook everything for 30 minutes on a high heat and top with the remaining sauce prior to serving.

TASTY CHICKEN TERIYAKI

This recipe needs 15 minutes to prepare, 6 hours to cook and will make 4 servings.

Each serving contains
- Protein: 27 grams
- Carbs: 25 grams
- Fats: 2 grams
- Saturated Fats: 1 gram
- Sugar: 1.7 grams
- Fiber 7 grams
- Calories: 217
- Smart Points: 5

What to Use
- Ground black pepper (to taste)
- Brown sugar (.25 cups)
- Soy sauce (.5 cups)
- Yellow pepper (.5 sliced thin)
- Red bell pepper (.5 sliced thin)
- Garlic (2 cloves minced)
- Pineapple (16 oz. chopped)
- Chicken breast (1 lb. cubed)

What to Do
1. In a small bowl, combine the brown sugar, black pepper, garlic and soy sauce and mix well.
2. Add the chicken to the slow cooker before topping with the soy sauce mixture and the pineapple.
3. Cover the slow cooker and let it cook on a low setting for 6 hours, after 5 hours remove the lid to allow the sauce to thicken.

COCONUT CHICKEN CURRY

This recipe needs 10 minutes to prepare, 4 hours to cook and will make 4 servings.

Each serving contains

- Protein: 28 grams
- Carbs: 17 grams
- Fats: 9 grams
- Sat. Fats: 2.7 grams
- Sugar: 9 grams
- Fiber 3 grams
- Calories: 272
- Smart Points: 6

What to Use

- Ground black pepper (to taste)
- Sea salt (to taste)
- Cornstarch (1 T)
- Brown sugar (2 T)
- Curry paste (3 T)
- Lime juice (1 lime)
- Garlic cloves (5 minced)
- Coconut milk (15 oz.)
- Stir fry vegetables (16 oz.)
- Yellow onion (1 sliced thin)
- Chicken breast (1 lb. diced)

What to Do

1. Season chicken as desired before adding it to the slow cooker and covering it with the onion.
2. Combine the curry paste, sugar, garlic, lime juice and coconut milk in a bowl and mix well.
3. Add the results to the slow cooker and cook, covered, on a low setting for 5 hours.
4. When there is half an hour of cooking time remaining, mix in the vegetables as well as the cornstarch mixed with 1 T water.

GREAT CHICKEN ITALIANO

This recipe needs 15 minutes to prepare, 6 hours to cook and will make 6 servings.

Each serving contains

- Protein: 31 grams
- Carbs: 9 grams
- Fats: 3 grams
- Saturated Fats: 5.7 g
- Sugar: 3 grams
- Fiber 1 grams
- Calories: 225
- Smart Points: 5

What to Use

- Ground black pepper (to taste)
- Sea salt (to taste)
- Paprika (2 tsp.)
- Chicken broth (1 cup)
- White wine (1 cup)
- Light butter (1 T)
- Cream cheese (8 oz.)
- Italian dressing mix (1 packet)
- Portabella mushrooms (8 oz. sliced)
- Mushrooms (8 oz. sliced)
- Chicken breast (1.5 lbs.)

What to Do

1. Add the butter to a saucepan before placing it on the stove on top of a burner set to a medium heat and mix in the Italian dressing thoroughly.
2. Add in the chicken broth, wine and cream cheese and keep stirring until the cream cheese has melted.
3. Add the mushrooms to the slow cooker before seasoning the chicken and adding it in as well. Add all of the ingredients to a slow cooker and let them cook, covered, on a low setting for 6 hours.

SMART POINTS SLOW COOKER TACOS

This recipe needs 20 minutes to prepare, 6 hours to cook and will make 8 servings.

Each serving contains
- Protein: 19 grams
- Carbs: 15 grams
- Fats: 17 grams
- Saturated Fats: 2.1 gram
- Sugar: .5 grams
- Fiber 2 grams
- Calories: 288
- Smart Points: 8

What to Use
- 6 inch tortillas (8)
- Bay leaves (2)
- Ground black pepper (to taste)
- Thyme (.25 tsp. dried)
- Cilantro (1 cup chopped)
- Cayenne pepper (.25 tsp.)
- Cinnamon (.5 tsp.)
- Cumin (.5 tsp. ground)
- Chuck roast (2 lbs. beef, cubed)
- Garlic (8 cloves minced)
- Onion (1 chopped)
- Tomatoes (2 chopped)
- 2 jalapeno peppers (chopped, seeded)

- Oil (1 T)

What to Do

1. Add the oil to a skillet and place it on the stove over a burner set to a medium/high heat.
2. Add in the garlic as well as the onion, tomatoes and peppers and let them cook for 5 minutes before removing them from the pan and adding them to a blender with 1 tsp. salt and .5 cups water and blend well.
3. Add the results back into the skillet before mixing in the beef and turning the burner to medium and let it brown.
4. Mix in the cayenne pepper, cinnamon and cumin and let everything cook for an additional minute.
5. As this cooks, add 1.5 cups of water as well as the thyme and cilantro into the blender and blend well.
6. Add all of the ingredients to the slow cooker and let them cook, covered, on a low heat for 6 hours.
7. Discard the bay leaves prior to adding the ingredients to the tortillas and serving.

ONE-POT CHICKEN WITH POTATOES

This recipe needs 15 minutes to prepare, 6 hours to cook and will make 6 servings.

Each serving contains

- Protein: 40 grams
- Carbs: 17.5 grams
- Fats: 7 grams
- Saturated Fats: 2.8 g
- Sugar: 1.5 grams
- Fiber 2 grams
- Calories: 301
- Smart Points: 6

What to Use

- Ground black pepper (to taste)
- Sea salt (to taste)
- Paprika (1 tsp.)
- Worcesershire sauce (1 T)
- Cheddar cheese (1 cup low fat)
- Chicken broth (.3 cups)
- Cream of chicken soup (10.75 oz.)
- Potatoes (1 lb. wedged)
- Chicken breast (6 fillets)

What to Do

1. Season the potatoes as needed before adding them to the slow cooker and then do the same with the chicken fillets.
2. Combine the broth with the soup before adding it to the slow cooker. Cover the slow cooker and let it cook on a low heat for 6 hours.
3. Remove the potatoes and the chicken from the slow cooker, leaving the broth/soup mixture in the slow cooker. Add in the cheese as well as Worcestershire sauce, cover and let everything cook for 5 minutes on a high heat.
4. Add the results to the chicken prior to serving.

ROSEMARY CHICKEN WITH LEMON

This recipe needs 20 minutes to prepare, 6 hours to cook and will make 4 servings.

Each serving contains
- Protein: 30 grams
- Carbs: 0 grams
- Fats: 8 grams
- Saturated Fats: 1.6 gram
- Sugar: 9.5 grams
- Fiber 0 grams
- Calories: 300
- Smart Points: 8

What to Use
- Ground black pepper (to taste)
- Sea salt (to taste)
- Butter (2 T)
- Garlic powder (1 tsp.)
- Sage (2 tsp. ground)
- Rosemary (3 sprigs)
- Onion (1 wedged)
- Lemons (2 sliced)
- Whole chicken (giblets removed, cleaned)

What to Do
1. Ensure your broiler is heated.
2. Season the chicken cavity as needed before adding in the rosemary, 50 percent of the onion wedges and 1 lemon.
3. Add the chicken to a roasting pan before coating it in utter and seasoning the outside as needed as well.
4. Place the pan in the oven and let the chicken cook for 8 minutes
5. Add all of the ingredients to a slow cooker and let them cook, covered, on a low setting for 6 hours.

CHICKEN AND DUMPLINGS

This recipe needs 15 minutes to prepare, 6 hours to cook and will make 6 servings.

Each serving contains
- Protein: 21 grams
- Carbs: 43 grams
- Fats: 5 grams
- Saturated Fats: 2 grams
- Sugar: 0 grams
- Fiber 3.5 grams
- Calories: 321
- Smart Points: 8

What to Use
- Ground black pepper (to taste)
- Sea salt (to taste)
- Chicken soup (10.75)
- Chicken broth (2 cups)
- Bouillon cube (1 chicken)
- Onion powder (2 tsp.)
- Thyme (2 tsp. dried)
- Reduced fat milk (.6 cups)
- Baking mix (2 cups)
- Celery (2 stalks diced)
- Carrots (2 diced)
- Potatoes (2 diced)
- Chicken breast (1 lb. boned, skinned)

What to Do
1. Add the bullion cube, celery stalks, carrots, potatoes and chicken to a slow cooker and season as needed.
2. Combine the thyme, onion powder, broth and soup together in a bowl and mix well before adding the results to the slow cooker and let them cook, covered, on a low setting for 6 hours.
3. Combine the milk with the baking mix together in a large bowl before adding the results, in 6 portions, to the top of the slow cooker. Turn the slow cooker heat to high and let everything cook an additional half hour.
4. You will know the dumplings are finished when you can stick a toothpick into one and it comes out clean. Don't forget to remove the lid from the slow cooker slightly to give the steam some place to go.

TORTILLA SOUP WITH CHICKEN

This recipe needs 10 minutes to prepare, 6 hours to cook and will make 6 servings.

Each serving contains

- Protein: 26 grams
- Carbs: 36 grams
- Fats: 2.8 grams
- Saturated Fats: .5 grams
- Sugar: 6 grams
- Fiber 7 grams
- Calories: 266
- Smart Points: 6

What to Use

- Ground black pepper (to taste)
- Sea salt (to taste)
- Garlic (4 cloves minced)
- Cumin (1 T0
- Chili powder (1 T)
- Chicken broth (2 cups)
- Tomatoes (28 oz. diced)
- Green chilies (4 oz. diced)
- Corn (15 oz. canned, rinsed, drained)
- Black beans (15 oz.)
- White beans (15 oz.)
- Red onion (1 diced)
- Chicken breast (1 lb. boned, skinned)

What to Do

1. Add all of the ingredients to a slow cooker and let them cook, covered, on a low setting for 6 hours.

SPICY SLOW COOKER CHICKEN

This recipe needs 10 minutes to prepare, 6 hours to cook and will make 6 servings.

Each serving contains
- Protein: 33 grams
- Carbs: 9.5 grams
- Fats: 4.5 grams
- Saturated Fats: 9.5 grams
- Sugar: 7.25 grams
- Fiber 1 grams
- Calories: 266
- Smart Points: 5

What to Use
- Ground black pepper (to taste)
- Sea salt (to taste)
- Rice vinegar (3 T)
- Soy sauce (.3 cups)
- Tomato paste (.25 cups)
- Honey (2 T)
- Sriracha sauce (.25 cups)
- Sesame oil (1 T)
- Garlic (4 cloves minced)
- Chicken breast (2 lbs. boned, skinned)

What to Do
1. Slice the chicken into strips.
2. In a small bowl, combine the rice vinegar, soy sauce, tomato paste, honey, sriracha sauce, sesame oil and garlic together and mix well before pouring onto the chicken and coating well.
3. Cover the slow cooker, set it to a low heat and let it cook for six hours.

CHICKEN NOODLE SOUP

This recipe needs 10 minutes to prepare, 6 hours to cook and will make 8 servings.

Each serving contains

- Protein: 6 grams
- Carbs: 60 grams
- Fats: 3 grams
- Saturated Fats: 1.5 g
- Sugar: 2 grams
- Fiber 15 grams
- Calories: 160
- Smart Points: 5

What to Use
- Ground black pepper (to taste)
- Sea salt (to taste)
- Parsley (.25 cups chopped)
- Lemon juice (.5 lemons)
- Egg noodles (4 oz.)
- Dill (1 tsp. dried)
- Rosemary (.5 tsp. dried)
- Thyme (1 tsp. dried)
- Garlic (2 cloves minced)
- Yellow onion (chopped fine)
- Celery (3 stalks chopped)
- Carrots (3 chopped)

What to Do
1. Add the dried dill, rosemary, thyme, garlic, onion, celery, carrots, broth, olive oil and chicken breast to a slow cooker and let them cook, covered, on a low setting for 6 hours.
2. Remove the chicken from the slow cooker before adding in the egg noodles, lemon juice and parsley and letting them cook on a low heat for 10 minutes.
3. Top the chicken with the results from the slow cooker prior to serving.

SLOW COOKED PORK CHILI

This recipe needs 15 minutes to prepare, 6 hours to cook and will make 8 servings.

Each serving contains
- Protein: 27 grams
- Carbs: 36 grams
- Fats: 3 grams
- Saturated Fats: 2.5 grams
- Sugar: 0 grams
- Fiber 5 grams
- Calories: 199
- Smart Points: 4

What to Use
- Ground black pepper (to taste)
- Sea salt (to taste)
- Cilantro (.25 cups chopped)
- Lime juice (1 lime)
- Cumin (1 T)
- Chili powder (1 T)
- Oregano (1 T)
- Garlic (2 cloves minced)
- Black beans (15 oz. rinsed, drained)
- Green chilies (8 oz. diced)
- Tomatoes (28 oz. diced)
- Onion (1 chopped fine)
- Pork tenderloin (1.5 lbs. cubed, fat removed)

What to Do
1. Prepare your slow cooker by coating it in cooking spray to prevent anything from sticking.
2. Start by placing the onions on the bottom of the slow cooker, followed by the pork, then the garlic, then the beans, green chilies and tomatoes. Top with spice and lime juice and mix well.
3. Let all of the ingredients cook, covered, on a low setting for 6 hours.
4. Top with cilantro prior to serving.

BLACK BEAN ENCHILADAS & SPINACH

This recipe needs 15 minutes to prepare, 3 hours to cook and will make 8 servings.

Each serving contains
- Protein: 26 grams
- Carbs: 30 grams
- Fats: 5 grams
- Saturated Fats: 3 grams
- Sugar: 7 grams
- Fiber 10 grams
- Calories: 217
- Smart Points: 7

What to Use
- Ground black pepper (to taste)
- Sea salt (to taste)
- Lime juice (1 lime)
- Chili powder (1 tsp.)
- Coriander (1 tsp. ground)
- Cumin (1 tsp. ground)
- Sharp cheddar cheese (1.5 cups shredded)
- Sour cream (.5 cups)
- Salsa Verde (24 oz.)
- Whole wheat tortilla (8)
- Corn (1 cup)
- Black beans (15 oz. rinsed, drained)
- Spinach (16 oz. frozen, thawed, squeezed)

What to Do

1. Place half the total number of black beans in a large bowl and mash them prior to adding in the pepper, salt, lime juice, chili powder, coriander, cumin, other black beans, corn and spinach and mix well.
2. Add half of the salsa to the slow cooker before adding the bean mixture to each tortilla and rolling tightly. Ideally all of the rolled tortillas will fit in a single layer in the slow cooker.
3. Add in the rest of the salsa along with the cheese and let everything cook, covered, on a low setting for 3 hours.
4. Top with jalapenos, onions, cilantro and sour cream prior to serving.

PULLED PORK AND CHEESE SANDWICH

This recipe needs 15 minutes to prepare, 7 hours to cook and will make 6 servings.

Each serving contains

- Protein: 27 grams
- Carbs: 34 grams
- Fats: 6.5 grams
- Saturated Fats: 5 grams
- Sugar: 2 grams
- Fiber 4 grams
- Calories: 315
- Smart Points: 8

What to Use
- Ground black pepper (to taste)
- Sea salt (to taste)
- Italian dressing mix (1 packet)
- Garlic (4 cloves minced)
- Basil (1 cup)
- Goat cheese (5 oz.)
- Spinach (14 oz. frozen, thawed)
- Red peppers (12 oz. chopped, drained, roasted)
- Pork roast (1 lb.)
- Sandwich rolls (6)

What to Do
1. Add the roast to the slow cooker before coating it in the garlic as well as the Italian dressing and seasoning as desired. Cook, covered, on a low setting for 7 hours.
2. Shred the pork and add in the spinach as well as the red peppers and let it cook for an additional 2 hours.
3. Toast the rolls and top with goat cheese before assembling the sandwiches.

ZUPPA TOSCANA SOUP

This recipe needs 15 minutes to prepare, 6 hours and 30 minutes to cook and will make 6 servings.

Each serving contains

- Protein: 14 grams
- Carbs: 20 grams
- Fats: 9.5 grams
- Saturated Fats: 4 grams
- Sugar: 5 grams
- Fiber 2 grams
- Calories: 212
- Smart Points: 6

What to Use

- Pork sausage (1 lb.)
- Potatoes (1 lb. diced, peeled)
- Garlic (4 cloves minced)
- Red pepper flakes (1 pinch)
- Ground black pepper (to taste)
- Sea salt (to taste)
- Half and half (1 cup)
- Whole wheat flower (2 T)
- Spinach leaves (3 cups)
- Chicken stock (3 cups)
- Onion (1 medium diced, peeled)

What to Do

1. The onion, garlic, potatoes and sausage to the slow cooker and let them cook, covered, on a low setting for 6 hours.
2. Combine the half and half with the flower in a mixing bowl before adding the results to the slow cooker before mixing in the spinach and combining thoroughly.
3. Cover the slow cooker, turn the heat to high and let it cook for 30 minutes more.
4. Season as desired prior to serving.

SPICY PULLED PORK

This recipe needs 10 minutes to prepare, 4 hours to cook and will make 6 servings.

Each serving contains
- Protein: 34.6 grams
- Carbs: 5 grams
- Fats: 3.6 grams
- Saturated Fats: 1 gram
- Sugar: 4.8 grams
- Fiber 7.7 grams
- Calories: 190
- Smart Points: 5

What to Use
- Apple cider vinegar (1 T)
- Chicken broth (1 cup)
- Garlic cloves (4 minced)
- Onion (1 diced)
- Pork tenderloin (2 lbs.)
- Coriander (.25 tsp.)
- Cinnamon (.25 tsp.)
- Pepper (.5 tsp.)
- Oregano (1 tsp.)
- Cumin (1 tsp. ground)
- Salt (1 tsp.)
- Chili powder (1 tsp.)
- Paprika (1 T)

What to Do
1. In a small bowl, combine the paprika, chili powder, salt, cumin, oregano, pepper, cinnamon and coriander together and mix well before applying the results to the whole of the pork tenderloin and rubbing well.
2. Add the pork to the slow cooker before adding in the onion and the garlic before covering everything with the chicken broth mixed together with the apple cider vinegar.
3. Cover the slow cooker and set it to a low heat before letting it cook for 6 hours.
4. Ensure your broiler is preheated
5. After the pork has finished cooing, shred it using a pair of forks before placing it in a baking tray and broiling it for 3 minutes to give it a crispy top layer.

TENDER BEEF STROGANOFF

This recipe needs 5 minutes to prepare, 6 hours to cook and will make 6 servings.

Each serving contains

- Protein: 20 grams
- Carbs: 15 grams
- Fats: 8 grams
- Saturated Fats: 3 grams
- Sugar: 6 grams
- Fiber 0 grams
- Calories: 216
- Smart Points: 7

What to Use

- Ground black pepper (to taste)
- Sea salt (to taste)
- Onion soup mix (1.25 oz.)
- Sour cream (16 oz.)
- Cream of mushroom soup (10.75 oz.)
- Ground beef (1 lb.)

What to Do

1. Place a skillet on the stove on top of a burner set to a high/medium heat before adding in the garlic, onion and beef and letting the beef brown.
2. Add the beef into the slow cooker before combining the other ingredients in a bowl and then adding them in on top.
3. Cover the slow cooker and let it cook on a low heat for 6 hours.

TASTY BEEF BURGUNDY

This recipe needs 15 minutes to prepare, 6 hours to cook and will make 6 servings.

Each serving contains
- Protein: 12 grams
- Carbs: 42 grams
- Fats: 9 grams
- Saturated Fats: 3.2 grams
- Sugar: 7 grams
- Fiber 0 grams
- Calories: 324
- Smart Points: 13

What to Use
- Ground black pepper (to taste)
- Sea salt (to taste)
- Egg noodles (3 cups cooked)
- Bay leaf (1)
- Mushroom (8 oz. sliced)
- Thyme (.5 tsp.)
- Onion (16 oz. chopped)
- Tomato paste (2 T)
- Red win e(.5 cups)
- Beef broth (10 oz.)
- All-purpose flour (.3 cups)
- Garlic (1 clove minced)
- Round steak (2 lbs. cubed)

What to Do

1. Place a skillet on the stove on top of a burner set to a high/medium heat. Add in the steak and let it brown before adding it to the slow cooking.
2. Add the garlic and onion to the skillet and coat the skillet using cooking spray before letting them cook 5 minutes. Add in the flour and cook an additional minute.
3. Add the rest of the ingredients to the skillet before adding it all to the slow cooker. Cover the slow cooker, turn it to a high heat and let it cook for an hour prior to turning the heat to low and cooking an additional 5 hours.
4. Remove the bay leaf and serve with the egg noodles.

BEAN SOUP WITH PORK SAUSAGE

This recipe needs 15 minutes to prepare, 8 hours to cook and will make 6 servings.

Each serving contains
- Protein: 19 grams
- Carbs: 31 grams
- Fats: 5 grams
- Saturated Fats: 5 grams
- Sugar: 3.5 grams
- Fiber 8 grams
- Calories: 240
- Smart Points: 6

What to Use
- Pork kielbasa (12 oz. sliced)
- Basil (1 tsp.)
- Dry red wine (.5 cups)
- Tomatoes (14.5 oz.)
- Northern beans (15.5 oz.)
- Red kidney beans (15.5 oz.)
- Vegetable broth (3 cups)
- Kale (.5 bunch leaves chopped, stems removed)
- Celery (1 stalk chopped)
- Carrot (1 chopped rough, peeled)
- Onion (1 chopped)
- Garlic (2 cloves minced)

What to Do
1. Add all of the ingredients, save the parmesan cheese, to the slow cooker and let them cook, covered, on a low setting for 8 hours.
2. Add the parmesan cheese prior to serving.

SLOW COOKER PORK POT ROAST

This recipe needs 10 minutes to prepare, 6 hours to cook and will make 8 servings.

Each serving contains
- Protein: 21 grams
- Carbs: 4 grams
- Fats: 12 grams
- Saturated Fats: 1 gram
- Sugar: 3 grams
- Fiber 0 grams
- Calories: 214
- Smart Points: 5

What to Use
- Pork shoulder roast (2 lbs.)
- Honey (1 T)
- Worcestershire sauce (1 T)
- Balsamic vinegar (.3 cups)
- Vegetable broth (.3 cups)
- Red pepper flakes (.5 tsp.)

What to Do
1. Season the pork prior to adding it to the slow cooker.
2. Combine the Worcestershire sauce with the vinegar as well as the broth before adding the

results to the top of the pork. Cover the slow cooker and let it cook on a low heat for 6 hours.
3. Remove the pork from the slow cooker and shred it before returning it to the slow cooker.
4. Plate the pork and top with sauce prior to serving.

CONCLUSION

Weight Watchers is one of the best diet pans that you can choose to go on. It is easy to follow and you are going to love how much good food you are able to enjoy while losing weight. I also love the fact that Weight Watchers is really paying attention to the science behind healthier foods being better for our bodies.

While some of the other diet plans that you may have tried in the past focused too much on telling you a long list of foods that you weren't allowed to eat, Weight Watchers allows you to live life and eat good foods all at the same time.

So take a look through this guidebook and find out just how easy and tasty the Weight Watchers diet can be!

Anna Kaiser

CPSIA information can be obtained
at www.ICGtesting.com
Printed in the USA
BVOW06s1144100118
504972BV00007B/34/P

9 781983 585272